Essentials of Environmental Public Health Science

Essentials of Environmental Public Health Science
A handbook for field professionals

Edited by

Naima Bradley
Henrietta Harrison
Greg Hodgson
Robie Kamanyire
Andrew Kibble
Virginia Murray

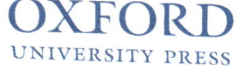

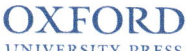

Great Clarendon Street, Oxford, OX2 6DP,
United Kingdom

Oxford University Press is a department of the University of Oxford.
It furthers the University's objective of excellence in research, scholarship,
and education by publishing worldwide. Oxford is a registered trade mark of
Oxford University Press in the UK and in certain other countries

© Oxford University Press 2014

The moral rights of the author have been asserted

First Edition published in 2014

All rights reserved. No part of this publication may be reproduced, stored in
a retrieval system, or transmitted, in any form or by any means, without the
prior permission in writing of Oxford University Press, or as expressly permitted
by law, by licence or under terms agreed with the appropriate reprographics
rights organization. Enquiries concerning reproduction outside the scope of the
above should be sent to the Rights Department, Oxford University Press, at the
address above

You must not circulate this work in any other form
and you must impose this same condition on any acquirer

Published in the United States of America by Oxford University Press
198 Madison Avenue, New York, NY 10016, United States of America

British Library Cataloguing in Publication Data
Data available

Library of Congress Control Number: 2013945736

ISBN 978-0-19-968288-1

Oxford University Press makes no representation, express or implied, that the
drug dosages in this book are correct. Readers must therefore always check
the product information and clinical procedures with the most up-to-date
published product information and data sheets provided by the manufacturers
and the most recent codes of conduct and safety regulations. The authors and
the publishers do not accept responsibility or legal liability for any errors in the
text or for the misuse or misapplication of material in this work. Except where
otherwise stated, drug dosages and recommendations are for the non-pregnant
adult who is not breast-feeding

Links to third party websites are provided by Oxford in good faith and
for information only. Oxford disclaims any responsibility for the materials
contained in any third party website referenced in this work.

Preface

Virginia Murray
Naima Bradley

With the advent of Public Health England (PHE), established on 1 April 2013 as an executive agency of the Department of Health, a wealth of specialist public health expertise, knowledge, and capability has been brought together into a single public health service that was, until then, distributed across a wide range of organisations and functions.

As a new national authoritative voice and expert service provider for public health, PHE undertakes the following functions:

- To protect and improve the nation's health and wellbeing, and tackle health inequalities so that the poorest and most poorly benefit most.
- To provide a nationwide, integrated public health service, supporting people to make healthier choices. It provides expertise, information, and intelligence to public health teams based in local authorities and the NHS to secure the biggest improvements in the public's health.
- To provide an integrated health protection service to ensure that everyone is protected from threats to their health from infectious disease and environmental hazards such as radiation, chemicals, and poisons.

PHE also has responsibilities across all UK countries for some functions related to radiation protection and chemical and other environmental hazards.

There is a continuing need for specialist training in environmental public health for staff in PHE and other agencies, including local authority environmental and public health professionals, and emergency planners and responders. PHE supports the need for the development of a comprehensive and structured national approach to education and training within the framework of continuing professional development and a national scheme of accredited Master's level modules and programmes in the areas of health protection and wider public health.

Spiby (2006) developed a model of core competencies required of those working in environmental public health that reflected the need for a 'coming together of the knowledge and skills base of environmental science, public health, clinical toxicology and environmental epidemiology'. Two main domains of competency were recognised:

1. Specialist environmental public health knowledge and skills
2. Generic organisational skills.

The first domain contained a number of areas of competency including toxicology, environmental public health, environmental epidemiology, and risk assessment and risk management.

The need for this book

In developing an 'Essentials of Environmental Public Health' Science training module, it became clear that there was no single suitable text for students coming from a variety of specialist backgrounds.

Intended audience

This book, a companion to the recently published *Essentials of Toxicology for Health Protection* (2012) and *Essentials of Environmental Epidemiology for Health Protection* (2012), is aimed at a wide range of professionals working in environmental public health, including health protection consultants, specialists, and trainees, public health practitioners, environmental health practitioners, environmental scientists, and staff of the emergency services, the water and waste industries, and other industrial and regulatory bodies.

It is assumed that most readers will be graduates with a good knowledge of public health sciences and an ability to carry out public health risk assessments. The practical nature of this book makes it a valuable tool for field practitioners who require an applied understanding of the essentials of environmental public health science.

Reference

Spiby, J. (2006). Developing competencies in environmental public health. *Chemical Hazards and Poisons Report*, **6**, 57–59. Health Protection Agency.

Acknowledgements

The editors wish to acknowledge the input from all the participants of the 'Essentials of Environmental Public Health' Science course over recent years. Their suggestions have assisted in preparing this book in a form most appropriate, relevant, and useful for future participants and other health professionals from a variety of disciplines.

We owe a special debt of thanks to Alec Dobney and Karen Hogan for their invaluable editorial support.

Contents

Abbreviations *xi*

Contributors *xv*

1 Introduction to *Essentials of Environmental Public Health Science* *1*
Naima Bradley and Alec Dobney

2 Physicochemical properties *9*
Nicholas Brooke

3 Key concepts and framework for investigation *20*
Camilla Ghiassee, Graham Urquhart, Raquel Duarte-Davidson, Jo Wilding, Charlotte Landeg-Cox, and Allister Gittins

4 Air pollution and public health *57*
Adrienne Dunne, Laura Mitchem, Jo Wilding, and Andrew Kibble

5 Water and public health *90*
Gary Lau, Stephen Robjohns, Frances Pollitt, Meera Cush, and Britta Gadeberg

6 Contaminated land and public health *115*
Yolande Macklin, Kerry Foxall, Paul Harold, Louise Uffindell, Sian Morrow, and George Kowalczyk

7 Waste management and public health *146*
Peter Lamb, Yolande Macklin, Andy McParland, and Greg Hodgson

8 Emerging issues *175*
Robie Kamanyire, Graham Urquhart, and Lorraine Stewart

Index of Statutes *198*

Subject Index *200*

Abbreviations

2-EDD	2-ethyl-5,5-dimethyl-1,3-dioxane	COC	Committee on carcinogenicity of chemicals in food, consumer products and the environment
2-EMD	2-ethyl-4-methyl-1,3-dioxolane		
AD	Anaerobic digestion	COMAH	Control of Major Accident Hazards
ADE	Average Daily Exposure	COMEAP	Committee on the Medical Effects of Air Pollutants
ADI	Acceptable daily intake		
AHVLA	Animal Health and Veterinary Laboratories Agency	CONTAM	Panel on Contaminants in the Food Chain
APC	Air pollution control	COPD	Chronic obstructive pulmonary disease
ALARP	As low as reasonably practicable		
AQEG	Air Quality Expert Group	COSHH	Control of Substances Hazardous to Health
AQMA	Air quality management area		
ATSDR	Agency for Toxic Substances and Disease Registry	COT	Committee on toxicity of chemicals in food, consumer products and the environment
ATT	Advanced Thermal Treatment		
AURN	Automatic Urban and Rural Network	CRCE	Centre for Radiation, Chemical and Environmental Hazards
BaP	Benzo[a]pyrene	CSDH	Commission on Social Determinants of Health
BAT	Best Available Techniques		
BEC	Biomass Energy Centre	CSM	Conceptual site model
BPA	Bisphenol A	DALY	Disability-adjusted life years
BGS	British Geological Survey	DAQI	Daily Air Quality Index
BMD	Benchmark dose	DBP	Disinfection by-product
BMDL	95 per cent lower confidence limit of the BMD	DECC	Department of Energy and Climate Change
BRE	Buildings Research Establishment	Defra	Department for Environment, Food and Rural Affairs
BREFs	Best available techniques reference documents	DETR	Department of the Environment, Transport and the Regions
BWA	Boil water advisory	DH	Department of Health
CA	Competent authority	DND	Do not use for drinking or cooking
CAS	Chemical Abstract Service	DNU	Do not use for drinking, cooking, or washing
CHEMET	Chemical Meteorology		
CHP	Combined heat and power	DQRA	Detailed quantitative risk assessment
CLEA	Contaminated Land Exposure Assessment	DWI	Drinking Water Inspectorate
		DWINI	Drinking Water Inspectorate for Northern Ireland
CLG	Communities and Local Government		
CLRTAP	Convention on Long-Range Transboundary Air Pollution	DWQR	Drinking Water Quality Regulator (for Scotland)
		EA	Environment Agency
CMA	Calcium magnesium acetate	EAP	Environmental Action Programme

EBoDE	Environmental Burden of Disease in Europe	JECFA	Joint FAO/WHO Expert Committee on Food Additives
EC	European Council	LA	Local authority
ECEH-Bonn	European Centre for Environment and Health in Bonn	LACORS	Local Authorities Co-ordinators of for Regulatory Services
ECHI	European Community Health Indicators	LAQM	Local air quality management
		LAQN	London Air Quality Network
ECHIM	European Community Health Indicators Monitoring	LEZ	Low emission zone
		LOAEL	Lowest Observed Adverse Effect Level
EDC	Endocrine disrupting chemical		
EFSA	European Food Safety Authority	LOCOG	London Organising Committee of the Olympic and Paralympic Games
ELV	Emission limit value		
ENHIS	Environment and Health Information Systems	LOD	Limits of detection
		LPG	Liquid petroleum gas
EPA	Environmental Protection Agency (US)	MAQS	Mayor's Air Quality Strategy
		MBT	Mechanical Biological Treatment
EPR	Environmental Permitting Regulations	MCDA	Multi-criteria decision analysis
		MDI	Mean daily intake
EWC	European Waste Catalogue	MetHb	Methaemoglobin
FAQ	'Frequently asked questions'	MOU	Memorandum of Understanding
FSA	Food Standards Agency	MSW	Municipal solid waste
GAC	Granular activated carbon	MW	Molecular weight
GAC	Generic Assessment Criteria	NBC	Normal Background Concentration
GBD	Global Burden of Disease (Study)	NHS	National Health Service
GIS	Geographic information system	NICOLE	Network for Industrially Contaminated Land in Europe
GLA	Greater London Authority		
GP	General Practitioner	NIEA	Northern Ireland Environment Agency
GPS	Global positioning systems		
GQRA	Generic quantitative risk assessment	NLC	North Lincolnshire Council
HAA	Haloacetic acid	NOAEL	No observed adverse effect level
HAN	Haloacetonitrile	NOM	Natural organic matter
HCV	Health Criteria Value	NPPF	National Planning Policy Framework
HPA	Health Protection Agency		
HSE	Health and Safety Executive	NRW	Natural Resources Wales
IARC	International Agency for Research on Cancer	OECD	Organisation for Economic Cooperation and Development
ICT	Idiopathic copper toxicosis	OSHA	Occupational Safety and Health Administration
ID	Index dose		
IED	Industrial Emissions Directive	PAH	Polycyclic aromatic hydrocarbon
IGHRC	Interdepartmental Group on Health Risks from Chemicals	PCDD	Polychlorinated dibenzodioxin
		PCDF	Polychlorinated dibenzofuran
IM	infantile methaemoglobinaemia	PCT	Primary Care Trust
IOC	International Olympic Committee	PFOS	Perfluorooctane sulfonic acid
IPC	Integrated Pollution Control	PHE	Public Health England
IPCS	International Programme on Chemical Safety	PHW	Public Health Wales
		PIE	PHYDADES Intelligent Energy

PM	Particulate matter	TCDD	2,3,7,8-tetracholoro-dibenzo-para-dioxin
POD	Point of departure	TDI	Tolerable daily intake
PPE	Personal protective equipment	TDSI	Tolerable daily soil intake
PRA	Preliminary risk assessment	TDU	Thermal desorption unit
QC	Quality control	THM	Trihalomethane
RBCA	Risk Based Corrective Action	UK-AIR	UK Air Information Resource
REACH	Registration, Evaluation, Authorisation and restriction of Chemicals	UKAS	UK Accreditation Service
		UNECE	United Nations Economic Commission for Europe
RISC	Risk Integrated Software for Clean-ups	UNIPHE	Use of sub-national indicators to improve public health in Europe
RPG	Regional priority goal		
RSC	Royal Society of Chemistry	VOC	Volatile organic compound
SAICM	Strategic Approach to International Chemicals Management	VP	Vapour pressure
		WDF	Waste-derived fuel
SCR	Selective catalytic reduction	WFD	Waste Framework Directive
SEERAD	Scottish Executive Environmental and Rural Affairs Department	WHO	World Health Organization
		WID	Waste Incineration Directive
SEPA	Scottish Environment Protection Agency	WMU	Water Management Unit
		WTW	Water treatment works
SG	Statutory Guidance	WWTW	Waste water treatment works
SGV	Soil Guideline Value	YLD	Years lived with disability
SPOSH	Significant possibility of significant harm	YLL	Years of life lost (due to premature mortality)
SSAC	Site specific assessment criteria		
SSBRA	Site-specific bioaerosol risk assessment		

Contributors

Editors

Dr Naima Bradley
Head of Department, Environmental Hazards and Emergencies
Centre for Radiation, Chemical and Environmental Hazards
Public Health England, UK

Henrietta Harrison
Head of Unit (Chilton/Bristol) – Environmental Hazards and Emergencies Department
Centre for Radiation, Chemical and Environmental Hazards
Public Health England, UK

Greg Hodgson
Head of Unit (Nottingham/Newcastle) – Environmental Hazards and Emergencies Department
Centre for Radiation, Chemical and Environmental Hazards
Public Health England, UK

Robie Kamanyire
Head of Unit (London) – Environmental Hazards and Emergencies Department
Centre for Radiation, Chemical and Environmental Hazards
Public Health England, UK

Andrew Kibble
Operations Manager
Centre for Radiation, Chemical and Environmental Hazards (Wales)
Public Health England, UK

Professor Virginia Murray
Head of Extreme Events and Health Protection Section
Centre for Radiation, Chemical and Environmental Hazards
Public Health England, UK

Assistant editors

Alec Dobney
Head of Unit (Birmingham/Manchester) – Environmental Hazards and Emergencies Department
Centre for Radiation, Chemical and Environmental Hazards
Public Health England, UK

Karen Hogan
Unit Administrator
Environmental Hazards and Emergencies Department (London Unit)
Centre for Radiation, Chemical and Environmental Hazards
Public Health England, UK

Contributors

Nicholas Brooke
Environmental Public Health Scientist
Environmental Hazards and Emergencies Department (London Unit)
Centre for Radiation, Chemical and Environmental Hazards
Public Health England, UK

Dr Meera Cush
Toxicologist
Toxicology Department
Centre for Radiation, Chemical and Environmental Hazards
Public Health England, UK

Alec Dobney
Head of Unit (Birmingham/Manchester) –
Environmental Hazards and Emergencies
Department
Centre for Radiation, Chemical and
Environmental Hazards
Public Health England, UK

Prof Raquel Duarte-Davidson
Head of International Research and
Development Group
Environmental Assessment Department
Centre for Radiation, Chemical and
Environmental Hazards
Public Health England, UK

Adrienne Dunne
Specialist Environmental Public Health
Scientist
Environmental Hazards and Emergencies
Department (London Unit)
Centre for Radiation, Chemical and
Environmental Hazards
Public Health England, UK

Kerry Foxall
Toxicologist
Toxicology Department
Centre for Radiation, Chemical and
Environmental Hazards
Public Health England, UK

Britta Gadeberg
Senior Toxicologist
Toxicology Department
Centre for Radiation, Chemical and
Environmental Hazards
Public Health England, UK

Camilla Ghiassee
Environmental Public Health Scientist
Environmental Hazards and Emergencies
Department (London Unit)
Centre for Radiation, Chemical and
Environmental Hazards
Public Health England, UK

Allister Gittins
Environmental Public Health Scientist
Environmental Hazards and Emergencies
Department (Chilton/Bristol Unit)
Centre for Radiation, Chemical and
Environmental Hazards
Public Health England, UK

Paul Harold
Environmental Public Health Scientist
Centre for Radiation, Chemical and
Environmental Hazards (Wales)
Public Health England, UK

George Kowalczyk
Regional Toxicologist
Environmental Hazards and Emergencies
Department (Birmingham/Manchester
Unit)
Centre for Radiation, Chemical and
Environmental Hazards
Public Health England, UK

Peter Lamb
Environmental Public Health Scientist
Environmental Hazards and Emergencies
Department (London Unit)
Centre for Radiation, Chemical and
Environmental Hazards
Public Health England, UK

Charlotte Landeg-Cox
Environmental Public Health Scientist
Environmental Hazards and Emergencies
Department (Chilton/Bristol Unit)
Centre for Radiation, Chemical and
Environmental Hazards
Public Health England, UK

Dr Gary Lau
Environmental Public Health Scientist
Environmental Hazards and Emergencies
Department (London Unit)
Centre for Radiation, Chemical and
Environmental Hazards
Public Health England, UK

Yolande Macklin
Environmental Public Health Scientist
Environmental Hazards and Emergencies Department (Birmingham/Manchester Unit)
Centre for Radiation, Chemical and Environmental Hazards
Public Health England, UK

Andy McParland
Environmental Public Health Scientist
Environmental Hazards and Emergencies Department (Nottingham/Newcastle Unit)
Centre for Radiation, Chemical and Environmental Hazards
Public Health England, UK

Dr Laura Mitchem
Principal Environmental Public Health Scientist
Environmental Hazards and Emergencies Department (Birmingham/Manchester Unit)
Centre for Radiation, Chemical and Environmental Hazards
Public Health England, UK

Sian Morrow
Environmental Public Health Scientist
Environmental Hazards and Emergencies Department (Birmingham/Manchester Unit)
Centre for Radiation, Chemical and Environmental Hazards
Public Health England, UK

Frances Pollitt
Principal Toxicologist
Toxicology Department
Centre for Radiation, Chemical and Environmental Hazards
Public Health England, UK

Stephen Robjohns
Senior Toxicologist
Toxicology Department
Centre for Radiation, Chemical and Environmental Hazards
Public Health England, UK

Dr Lorraine Stewart
Principal Environmental Public Health Scientist
Environmental Hazards and Emergencies Department (Chilton/Bristol Unit)
Centre for Radiation, Chemical and Environmental Hazards
Public Health England, UK

Dr Louise Uffindell
Environmental Public Health Scientist
Environmental Hazards and Emergencies Department (Chilton/Bristol Unit)
Centre for Radiation, Chemical and Environmental Hazards
Public Health England, UK

Dr Graham Urquhart
Principal Environmental Public Health Scientist
Environmental Hazards and Emergencies Department (Chilton/Bristol Unit)
Centre for Radiation, Chemical and Environmental Hazards
Public Health England, UK

Dr Jo Wilding
Environmental Public Health Scientist
Environmental Hazards and Emergencies Department (Nottingham/Newcastle Unit)
Centre for Radiation, Chemical and Environmental Hazards
Public Health England, UK

Chapter 1

Introduction to *Essentials of Environmental Public Health Science*

Naima Bradley and Alec Dobney

> **Learning objectives**
>
> By the end of this chapter the reader will be able to:
> - understand the role of environmental public health
> - understand the relation between environmental epidemiology, toxicology, environmental science, and health protection.

Introduction

Essentials of Environmental Public Health Science is intended to be a course book for students, and a handbook for field professionals involved in responding to local environmental public health concerns. The book is not aimed solely at public health professionals within in the UK but also those further afield. It provides practical guidance on the technical aspects of environmental and public health investigations. The authors frequently provide practical, expert advice to a range of public health professionals and have been chosen for their knowledge, experience, and skills to compile this applied, evidence-based book. Much of the material in this book has been taught by the authors in Masters in Public Health programmes and at UK and international training seminars.

Environmental public health provides an interdisciplinary approach to the study of the direct and indirect impact of exposure to environmental hazards on the public's health and wellbeing. Assessing and addressing the risks of chemical, ionizing and non-ionizing radiation, and noise hazards requires a sound knowledge of toxicology, environmental epidemiology, environmental science, health risk assessment, and public health principles. Whilst radiation and noise are areas of study for environmental public health scientists, they are large topics in their own right warranting greater treatment than can be afforded in this book. As such, they are deemed to be outside the scope of this book.

The quality of the environment plays an important role in health and wellbeing. Worldwide, environmental hazards are responsible for nearly a quarter of the total burden of disease, although the nature of environmental risks varies in different socio-economic

Table 1.1 Deaths and DALYs attributable to five environmental risks, and to all five risks combined by region, 2004

Risk	World	Low and middle income	High income
Percentage of deaths			
Indoor smoke from solid fuels	3.3	3.9	0.0
Unsafe water, sanitation, hygiene	3.2	3.8	0.1
Urban outdoor air pollution	2.0	1.9	2.5
Global climate change	0.2	0.3	0.0
Lead exposure	0.2	0.3	0.0
All five risks	**8.7**	**9.6**	**2.6**
Percentage of DALYs			
Indoor smoke from solid fuels	2.7	2.9	0.0
Unsafe water, sanitation, hygiene	4.2	4.6	0.3
Urban outdoor air pollution	0.6	0.6	0.8
Global climate change	0.4	0.4	0.0
Lead exposure	0.6	0.6	0.1
All five risks	**8.0**	**8.6**	**1.2**

Reproduced from World Health Organization, *Global health risks: mortality and burden of disease attributable to selected major risks,* Copyright © 2009, with permission from the World Health Association, available at: http://www.who.int/healthinfo/global_burden_disease/GlobalHealthRisks_report_full.pdf.

groups. Table 1.1 shows the distribution of environmental mortality and the combined burden due to death and disability in a single index called the Disability-Adjusted Life Years (DALY). The DALY index allows comparison between risk factors or diseases (see Chapter 8).

Children are particularly vulnerable as their bodies are still developing, which means that their biological systems may be more susceptible to harm from environmental hazards; additionally, their exposures may be higher because they take in more food, water, and air per kilogram body weight than adults. The burden of disease amongst children due to environmental hazards has been estimated to be more than one third of the total burden of disease worldwide (Prüss-Üstün and Corvalán, 2006).

Unsustainable waste disposal, energy generation, transport, and land uses could impact significantly on the air, water, and land quality and thus on the public's health. Undertaking a comprehensive assessment of the risks to individuals from these activities is a complex task. Comprehensive health risk assessments not only consider people's exposure to individual substances released into the environment, but also take into account genetics, pre-existing diseases, socioeconomic factors, environmental and community conditions, and individual behaviour. This book will only consider a small element of the overall health risks, this being the risk to populations from exposure to chemical hazards.

An important concept in environmental public health is the difference between hazards and risks. Hazards have the potential to cause harm. Hazards can be natural (for example, flooding) or as a result of human activity (for example emissions from industry). They can be physical agents (for example noise), biological (for example bacteria), or chemical in origin. The risk is the likelihood of harm as a result of exposure to hazards. Risk is usually expressed as a ratio or percentage; for example, risk from chronic exposures is expressed as the lifetime risk, for example for carcinogens, a lifetime risk of 1 in 10^{-6} (one in a million) of developing cancer over the course of a lifetime is considered acceptable and is insignificant compared to the natural background lifetime cancer incidence rate of about 30 per cent. Public concern depends on how people view the risk, how it is communicated, and by whom. Communication plays a vital part in how people will accept the outcome of a risk assessment process. Environmental public health professionals use robust methodologies to identify hazards, assess their potential consequences, and characterise, identify, and prioritize risk management strategies. They must also acquire expertise and experience in communicating with members of the public, policy makers, other scientists, regulators, and businesses.

A simplified model for assessing risks is the source–pathway–receptor model. Information about a substance (source), its fate and behaviour in the environment (pathway), and the population at risk (receptor) is gathered, analysed, and assessed. A chemical's potential to cause harm will depend on the actual substance, its physicochemical properties, and its impact on the human body. Information on quantity and spatial distribution in air, water, and land can be gathered through a combination of sampling and dispersion modelling. This information can then be used to determine the likelihood of exposure to the substance in the population at risk. Further information on the potentially exposed population is needed to define particularly vulnerable people such as the young, elderly, and people with relevant pre-existing diseases.

As well as allowing public health professionals to tackle risk assessments for local environmental stressors, information on the source and environmental distribution of pollutants and their impact on health inform the development of environmental policy. There are many examples where environmental public health science has contributed to reducing harm from exposure to hazardous chemicals through environmental policy and legislation; for example, by removing lead from petrol, banning asbestos-containing materials, and setting health standards for priority pollutants in air and water. However, major challenges remain despite the improvement in our environment. For example, fine particles suspended in the atmosphere emitted from road transport and industry can cause serious health effects and there is no evidence of a safe level of exposure. Emissions from road transport accounted for around a quarter of the total $PM_{2.5}$ (particulate matter less than 2.5 μm in diameter) emissions. Despite a reduction of 72 per cent for $PM_{2.5}$ emissions between 1970 and 2011 in the UK, air pollution is still a major cause of ill-health as short- and long-term exposure can worsen respiratory and cardiovascular illness and increase mortality (Defra, 2012a). Particulate matter concentrations have changed little in the past 5 years (Defra, 2012b).

Although unlikely to be achievable, the total elimination of man-made fine particles would result in gains in life expectancy of 7–8 months (based on 2005 levels). This would make a greater impact than eliminating motor vehicle traffic accidents (1–3 months) or second-hand cigarette smoke (2–3 months). The UK annual health cost attributed to air pollution is £15 billion compared to the estimated health cost of obesity of £10 billion (Defra, 2010a).

As well as people's direct exposure to pollutants, identifying, understanding, and tackling environmental inequalities is important; therefore, socio-economic issues need to be considered. Environmental inequalities arise where deprived communities experience a poorer environmental quality. For example, a study comparing the spatial distribution of certain industrial sites in England and Wales against patterns of deprivation showed that regulated industries were clustered in areas near deprived populations (Walker et al., 2005). However, proximity to a pollution source doesn't necessarily mean that people living nearby are exposed to such high levels of pollutants that ill-health will be caused.

Defra's indicator on environmental equality (Defra, 2010b) shows that 0.2 per cent of people living in the least deprived areas in the UK may experience the 'least favourable' environmental conditions, compared to approximately 17 per cent of people living in the most deprived areas. People living in the most deprived communities will, on average, die 7 years earlier than people with higher socio-economic status. Creating and developing sustainable places and communities and strengthening the role and impact of ill-health prevention are two of the six main recommendations of the Marmott review (Marmott, 2010). In this fast-developing agenda of social justice and appetite for tackling environmental inequalities, environmental public health professionals can influence government policy and act as public health advocates at national, regional, or local level.

Environmental sciences and health protection

Environmental guideline parameters for water, air, or land quality, designed to protect human health, are based on our current understanding of environmental sciences including environmental chemistry, environmental toxicology, and epidemiological studies.

Information needed to reach evidence-based decisions on the control and management of chemicals in the environment is only available for a very few of the 71 million organic and inorganic substances in existence. In 2007, the EU adopted legislation on the Registration, Evaluation, Authorisation and restriction of Chemicals (REACH). One of the objectives of REACH is the protection of human health through better understanding of the intrinsic properties of chemical substances. REACH places the burden of proof on industry to demonstrate that a chemical can be used safely and it has explicit requirements for reproductive and developmental toxicity data on substances manufactured in or imported into the European Union at or above 10 metric tons/year. A review commissioned by the EU concluded that this legislation is beginning to deliver the intended benefits by, for example, removing some substances of very high concern from use. In the meantime, information already available on the toxicity of compounds is used by environmental public health scientists to assess and mitigate the risks posed by historical contamination (for example contaminated land from past industrial uses) and modern activities such as novel waste management and energy generation activities.

Environmental scientists and chemists study the interaction of chemicals in the environment, their persistence, chemical transformation, and biodegradation within one or more environmental compartments. Improvements in analytical techniques allow more accurate and precise measurement of individual pollutants within air, water, and land. Models, linked with geographic information systems (GIS), allow mapping of the spatial and temporal distributions of pollutants, thereby providing us with better visual information to refine the exposure assessment.

A chemical, either in its original form or through its degradation products, needs to be transferred by ingestion, inhalation, or dermal contact from the environment to a human being in order to cause harm; this is called the exposure phase. Once absorbed, the process by which the body deals with a toxic substance through distribution, accumulation, biotransformation, and elimination is known as toxicokinetics. Toxicodynamics describes the mechanism by which a toxic substance affects the site of action (cells in organs and so on) and produces a toxic effect. One of the key toxicological concepts is the dose–response assessment. It describes the relationship between the dose of a substance and the magnitude of its effect, thus linking the likelihood of a particular effect with a dose. Descriptions and practical examples of the way chemicals cause toxic effects can be found in *Essentials of Toxicology for Health Protection* (Baker et al., 2012).

Using information provided by toxicological studies about which substances are harmful to human health, and the mode of action and magnitude of the harm, environmental epidemiologists study the cause and distribution of disease and health-related events at the community level. Environmental epidemiologists focus on causes of diseases due to exposure to physical, biological, or chemical hazards in the external environment. Key environmental policy decisions, such as those relating to air quality, are often based on epidemiological studies. These play an important role in supplying the risk coefficients that are used in quantitative risk assessments.

In the UK, disease clusters caused by non-infectious environmental agents, defined as an unusually high number of similar cases in a given area, time period, or population, are thankfully rare. However, triggers such as persistent odours, unusual events (for example large fires), close proximity to a landfill or incinerator, or the perception that diseases such as cancers are prevalent in the community, can lead to complaints and allegations of disease clusters. Public health professionals deal with such allegations in a sympathetic and professional way. They gather information and document the subjective and objective health effects (medically diagnosed conditions will carry more weight than self-reported symptoms). They consider the biological plausibility of the claims (that is, whether or not the association is consistent with what is already known about the disease or the response to the exposure) and they gather information about the potential source, comparing environmental pollutant concentration with relevant health standards where they exist.

The decision to launch a full investigation depends on an assessment of the quality of the evidence. This requires a multi-disciplinary approach involving toxicologists, environmental public health scientists, environmental epidemiologists, and public health professionals. A more detailed description of cluster investigations and other epidemiological investigations and case studies can be found in *Essentials of Environmental Epidemiology for Health Protection* (Kreis et al., 2012).

Structure of the book

This book is designed to cover a wide range of environmental public health issues from a practitioner's perspective and bring together important aspects of environmental public health in one place. The book is aimed at a range of professional users, from the seasoned practitioner to those who have little experience of the technical aspects of environmental and health investigations.

Chapter 2 describes how the physicochemical properties of chemicals can be used to help predict potential environmental public health consequences and the way in which chemicals behave in the environment. The chapter defines common terms and outlines the way in which environmental public health scientists use tools, such as screening by physicochemical properties, to assist in the assessment of risks to health.

Chapter 3 describes some of the broad concepts of environmental public health and sets out the framework for investigation, including the principles of environmental legislation and risk assessment. It outlines how risk assessment involves an analysis of the consequences and probability that a hazard will result in adverse health effects under specific circumstances. The importance of risk perception and risk communication is highlighted as an aspect of environmental public health that cross-cuts many fields and disciplines. The practical applications of certain tools used in risk assessments, such as geographic information systems, are described. General principles of environmental sampling and monitoring, including methods of analysis and handling of accuracy and uncertainty, are explored. The key environmental models are summarised, along with their main limitations. There are also practical examples of using environmental sampling, monitoring, and modelling to inform environmental public health decisions and protect the population.

In Chapter 4, the importance of local, regional, national, and international sources of air pollution (primary and secondary) and new and emerging issues are discussed. The role of regulation and local air quality strategies is examined with case studies of local problems focussing on control and intervention measures used to improve areas of poor air quality. The health effects of important ambient air pollutants are discussed. The chapter uses case studies to highlight good practice and challenges in assessing the impact of air pollution on health, as well as key interventions and control measures to minimise individual and population exposures.

A general introduction to the importance of clean water to public health is provided in Chapter 5. The case studies address the public health implications of public and private water supplies. Key sources of pollution are considered, such as agricultural activities, and their impact on private drinking water supplies is explored.

Chapter 6 provides examples to enhance public health responders' knowledge of contaminated land and adaptation of risk assessment methodologies for evaluating hazards and protecting exposed communities. Case studies identify good practice and challenges in assessing the impact of soil pollution on health. The chapter discusses the fate and behaviour of common soil pollutants in different soil types and compares the behaviour of pollutants in water and air. Additionally, it highlights the unique challenges presented by contaminants in soil. Soil sorption properties (soil as a pollutant sink), residence times, and uptake into plants of pollutants such as heavy metals, polycyclic aromatic hydrocarbons (PAHs), and dioxins are described. The influence of pollutant behaviour on routes of exposure is discussed in terms of bioavailability and accessibility.

Wastes are controlled by wide-ranging and far-reaching regulatory frameworks. Chapter 7 introduces the concept of waste management and explains how the control of waste is a public health issue. It covers the development of waste regulation and explains current European and UK legislation. Different types of waste streams are described, along with emerging waste management technologies and their associated public health impacts and concerns. The chapter outlines the added value that public health professionals can bring to the regulation of waste management processes by supporting the regulation of waste, expanding the knowledge base, and developing the understanding of associated public health risks and risk perception.

Finally, Chapter 8 considers some of the key emerging issues for environmental public health, recognising that environmental pollution is an important contributory cause of the underlying burden of disease. The importance of tackling environmental inequalities and promoting environmental sustainability, along with the impact on global environmental change, is also discussed. The chapter also outlines the importance of tools to assess population health and target policies and interventions in order to protect health at local, regional, and national level. It describes techniques, such as 'horizon scanning', that assist public health professionals to identify and assess future threats or potential opportunities at an early stage and ensure health is protected.

At the beginning of each chapter of the book, key learning objectives are identified. Practical applications of environmental public health issues are illustrated with the inclusion of case studies to emphasise particular issues and reinforce the subject knowledge.

References

Defra (2010a). Air pollution: Action in a changing climate. Available at: https://www.gov.uk/government/uploads/system/uploads/attachment_data/file/69340/pb13378-air-pollution.pdf [Accessed 26 May 2013].

Defra (2010b). Measuring progress: Sustainable development indicators 2010. Available at: http://sd.defra.gov.uk/documents/MPSD2010.pdf [Accessed 26 May 2013].

Defra (2012a). UK emissions of air pollutants 1970 to 2011. Available at: https://www.gov.uk/government/uploads/system/uploads/attachment_data/file/82998/Emissions_of_air_pollutants_statistical_release_1970–2011.pdf [Accessed 26 May 2013].

Defra (2012b). Air quality statistics in the UK, 1987 to 2012. Available at: https://www.gov.uk/government/uploads/system/uploads/attachment_data/file/192277/Air_Qual_Statistics_final_release2012v2.pdf [Accessed 26 May 2013].

Marmott Review team (2010). Fair society, healthy lives: Strategic review of health inequalities in England post-2010. Available at: http://www.instituteofhealthequity.org/projects/fair-society-healthy-lives-the-marmot-review/fair-society-healthy-lives-full-report [Accessed 26 May 2013].

Prüss-Üstün, A. and Corvalán, C. (2006). Preventing disease through healthy environments. Towards an estimate of the environmental burden of disease. Available at: http://www.who.int/quantifying_ehimpacts/publications/preventingdisease.pdf [Accessed 26 May 2013].

Walker, G., Mitchell, G., Fairburn, J., and Smith, G. (2005). Industrial pollution and social deprivation: Evidence and complexity in evaluating and responding to environmental inequality. *Local Environment: The international journal of justice and sustainability*, **10**:4, 361–377. Available at: http://www.tandfonline.com/doi/abs/10.1080/13549830500160842 [Accessed 26 May 2013].

World Health Organization (2009). Global health risks: Mortality and burden of disease attributable to selected major risks. Available at: http://www.who.int/healthinfo/global_burden_disease/GlobalHealthRisks_report_full.pdf [Accessed 26 May 2013].

Further Reading

Ayres, J., Harrison, R., Nichols, G., and Maynard, R. (2010). *Environmental Medicine*. Edward Arnold, London.

Baker, D., Karalliedde, L., Murray, V. S. G., Maynard, R., and Parkinson, N. (Eds) (2012). 2nd ed. *Essentials of Toxicology and Health Protection: A handbook for field professionals*. Oxford University Press, Oxford.

Chemical Abstract Service (2013). CAS Registry 2013. Available at: http://www.cas.org/ [Accessed 26 May 2013].

Kreis, I., Busby, A., Leonardi, G., Meara, J., and Murray, V. S. G. (Eds) (2012). *Essentials of Environmental Epidemiology for Health Protection: A handbook for field professionals*. Oxford University Press, Oxford.

Chapter 2

Physicochemical properties

Nicholas Brooke

Learning objectives

By the end of this chapter the reader will be able to:
- understand a wide range of physicochemical properties including their interpretation and units of measurement
- understand how physicochemical properties affect the environmental behaviour of chemicals in air, land, and water
- understand how physicochemical properties affect the toxicity of a chemical and influence an environmental decontamination strategy.

Introduction

Industrial and technological developments have led to a continual expansion in the number of chemical compounds being synthesised (or isolated) and reported in the scientific literature. The Chemical Abstract Service (CAS) was formed in 1907 to collate and publish information on chemical substances. The CAS database now contains information on over 70 million chemicals (CAS, 2013).

Chemicals may occur as liquids, solids, or gases, and of those in use, many can cause acute or chronic toxic effects. Figure 2.1 illustrates the main human exposure routes. As it is not possible to determine the environmental behaviour or toxicity of every individual chemical, scientists use tools, including screening by physicochemical properties, to assist. This chapter aims to provide an overview of physicochemical properties and guidance on how they can be interpreted.

Environmental public health professionals may interpret a number of physicochemical properties when responding to chemical incidents. For those properties commonly utilised, a description of how it may influence environmental behaviour in water, soil, and air is provided. Examples are provided of how physicochemical properties can influence the absorption of chemicals via ingestion, skin contact, or inhalation leading to exposure and potential toxicity. Environmental decontamination or 'clean up' techniques may be undertaken to reduce or avert the exposure of people to chemical contamination in the

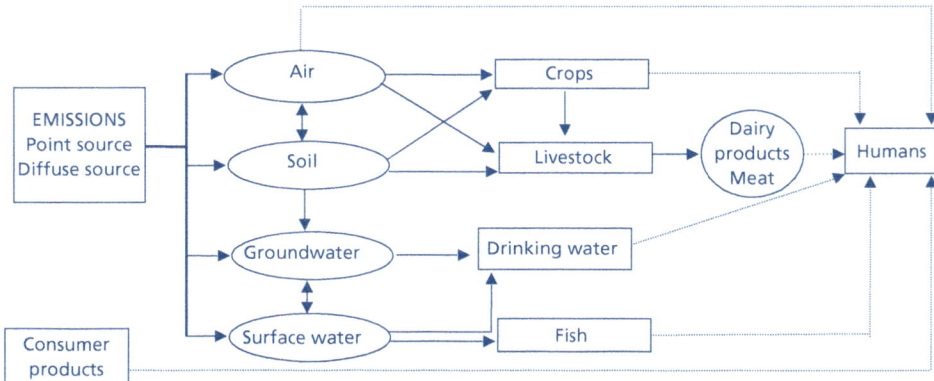

Fig. 2.1 Schematic representation of the main exposure routes for humans.

Reproduced from Institute for the Environment and Health, *A Screening Method for Ranking Chemicals by their Fate and Behaviour in the Environment and Potential Toxic Effects in Humans Following Non-occupational Exposure* (Web Report W14), Copyright © 2004, with permission from IEH, available from http://www.le.ac.uk/ieh/.

environment following a chemical release. Hence, for each physicochemical property, examples of appropriate decontamination techniques are also provided. A quick guide to how physicochemical properties may be interpreted is presented in Table 2.1, which was originally developed as part of the *UK Recovery Handbook for Chemical Incidents* (Wyke-Sanders et al., 2012) to consider environmental decontamination, but has been adapted further to consider toxicological endpoints. Less commonly used physicochemical properties are also contained within this table, including molecular weight and Henry's Law constant. Henry's Law gives an indication of how a chemical partitions between a solution and the air above it and hence the tendency for chemicals to move from a liquid or solid (for example soil) into the atmosphere.

Physicochemical properties

Physical form

Gases will generally disperse quickly once released in the environment, especially in outdoor areas. They present an inhalational hazard. Stable gases (for example helium or xenon) tend to have reversible asphyxiant or anaesthetic effects whereas reactive gases such as halogens (for example chlorine) are more likely to cause physical damage to the respiratory tract (Dahl, 1990).

Liquids will generally flow and spread in an environment according to gravity. They primarily represent a dermal contact hazard but volatile liquids such as acetone can also pose an additional risk via inhalation.

Solids are generally less mobile in the environment, although they can disperse in the form of dust, smoke, or fumes, especially during incidents involving fires. They can present a hazard when they have been ingested (often inadvertently), although if the individual

Table 2.1 Interpretation of physicochemical properties

Property	Description	Interpretation	
Vapour pressure (VP)	Units = Pascals (Pa) <1.3×10^{-4} Pa: Unlikely to volatilise Between 1.3×10^{-4} and 1.3 Pa: Increasing likelihood of volatilising >1.3 Pa: Likely to volatilise	High VP **Likely to:** Be an inhalational hazard Evaporate quickly Be contained by fixative coatings	Low VP **Unlikely to be:** An inhalational hazard Persistent
Vapour density	Air is assigned an arbitrary value of 1 and if a gas has a vapour density of <1.29, it will generally rise in air. If the vapour density is >1.29, the gas will generally sink.	D >1.29 **Likely to:** Remain close to the ground and pose a risk to inhabitants	D <1.29 **Likely to:** Rise and mix in air more easily but may accumulate in indoor ceiling spaces
Water solubility	Units: mg/l or ppm <10: Negligible solubility Between 10 and 1000: Increasing likelihood of solubilizing >1000: Likely to solubilise	High solubility **Likely to:** Contaminate groundwater Be decontaminated by water-based solutions Be mobile in the environment **Unlikely to:** Be volatilised	Low solubility **Likely to be:** Immobilised by adsorption **Unlikely to:** Be mobile in the environment Contaminate drinking water
Partition coefficient between water and octanol	Units = K_{ow} >1000: Likely to bioaccumulate. High Between 500 and 1000: Increasing likelihood of bioaccumulating <500: Unlikely to bioaccumulate. Low	High K_{ow} **Likely to:** Accumulate in fatty tissue Cross the blood-brain barrier Be absorbed across skin Permeate plastic pipes **Unlikely to be:** Decontaminated by water alone Mobile	Low K_{ow} **Likely to be:** Mobile Soluble **Unlikely to be:** Bioaccummulated
Persistence (water and air)	Units = T½ Median half-life | Water and air (days)	Soil (days)	Persistence
---	---	---
<0.042 (1 hour)	<5	Very short-lived
0.042–0.42	<15	Short-lived
0.42–4	<30	Moderately short-lived
4–40	30–100	Moderately persistent
>40	>100	Highly persistent		High persistence **Likely to:** Remain in relevant medium and result in exposure Be difficult to decontaminate **Unlikely to:** Be volatile Be reactive	Short persistence **Likely to be:** Volatile Reactive **Unlikely to:** Require decontamination

(continued)

Table 2.1 (continued) Interpretation of physicochemical properties

Property	Description	Interpretation	
Soil sorption	Interpretation (units = K_{OC}) >10,000: Likely to adsorb Between 1000 and 10,000: Increasing likelihood of adsorbing <1000: Unlikely to adsorb	High K_{OC} **Likely to be:** Adsorbed to soil Accumulated **Unlikely to be:** Mobile	Low K_{OC} **Likely to be:** Mobile **Unlikely to be:** Adsorbed
Specific gravity	Assuming a substance is insoluble in water: If the specific gravity is less than 1.0, it will float If greater than 1.0, it will sink	D >1 **Likely to:** Sink in water	D <1 **Likely to:** Form a surface film on water Potentially pose a hazard to recreational water users Be decontaminated using booms
Henry's Law constant	Units: Unitless or in Pa m³/mol where 1 Pa = 9.872 × 10⁻⁶ atm >1 × 10⁻⁴ Higher tendency to volatilise <1 × 10⁻⁴ Lower tendency to volatilise	High Hc **Likely to:** Have potential for volatilisation from water surfaces Result in exposure via inhalation	Low Hc **Likely to:** Have a low potential for volatilization Remain in solution
Molecular weight (MW)	Unit: g/mole *Substances heavier than 600 g/mole are unlikely to cross the blood-brain barrier Hydrophobic (see K_{ow}) substances with a low molecular weight are more likely to cross the blood-brain barrier	High MW **Likely to:** Have a low solubility in water	Low MW **Likely to:** Cross the blood-brain barrier or placenta Be absorbed and result in a toxic effect Be volatile

Adapted from Wyke-Sanders et al., *UK Recovery Handbook for Chemical Incidents*, Health Protection Agency, Copyright © 2012 with permission from the HPA, available from http://www.hpa.org.uk/Publications/RemediationAndEnvironmentalDecontamination/1205UKrecoveryhandbookforchemincidents and Department of the Environment, Transport and the Regions, *Environmental Sampling After a Chemical Accident*, The Stationery Office, London, UK, Copyright © 1999, licensed under the Open Government Licence v1.0.

particles are small enough they also pose an inhalational risk when dispersed as dust, fibres, or particulates, which often exert toxic effects via mechanical irritation.

Environmental decontamination

Absorbent materials such as sand or fuller's earth may be used to 'soak up' a liquid spillage. Impermeable barriers (for example temporary walls) may be used to limit the spread of a toxic gas or vapour following a chemical release (Wyke-Sanders et al., 2012). Solids may be decontaminated using methods such as wet wiping to remove dust, as was implemented after the 9/11 terrorist attacks (OSHA, 2002).

Vapour pressure

The vapour pressure is the saturation pressure exerted by vapours that are in equilibrium with their liquid or solid forms (RSC, 2013). In simple terms, it indicates how easily a substance evaporates.

The vapour pressure of a chemical is influenced by temperature. At higher temperatures, a liquid will release more vapour or turn into a gas. Some liquids are described as volatile and these liquids will have high vapour pressures even at ambient or low temperatures. Volatile chemicals are generally less persistent. The boiling point represents the temperature at which a liquid changes from the liquid state to a gaseous state (Dahl, 1990).

A high vapour pressure indicates that a chemical is likely to pose an inhalational hazard. Flammable chemicals with a high vapour pressure tend to create a hazardous atmosphere with an explosive risk.

Environmental decontamination

The use of fixative coatings (for example firefighting foam/specialised paints) can create a temporary or permanent barrier between the chemical and the surrounding air (Wyke-Sanders et al., 2012).

Vapour density

Vapour density is the density of a vapour in relation to that of a reference gas; air is the most often used reference gas. Gases that are lighter than air will usually disperse more widely in the environment, although they can become trapped in ceiling voids or spaces following an indoor release. Hence, volatile gases with a high vapour pressure that are also heavier than air can collect in low-lying spaces such as basements, cellars, or in holds of ships and are more likely to lead to exposure to the public in inhabitable areas (DETR, 1999).

Environmental decontamination

The use of appropriate ventilation by using fans and opening doors and windows facilitates the dispersal of gases or vapours that have accumulated within indoor areas.

Water solubility

Water solubility describes the tendency for chemicals to dissolve into water and reflects the amount of chemical that can dissolve in a known quantity of water. Water soluble chemicals are more likely to be leached from soil and migrate downwards to contaminate groundwater than chemicals with low solubility. Insoluble chemicals tend to separate to form a layer when mixed with water (DETR, 1999).

Water soluble chemicals, especially if persistent (that is slowly degraded or metabolised), may contaminate groundwater and lead to potential public exposure via the ingestion of contaminated drinking water.

Environmental decontamination

For water soluble chemicals, the decontamination of interior or exterior building surfaces may be primarily carried out with water-based cleaning methods such as steam cleaning or pressure hosing (Wyke-Sanders et al., 2012).

Partition coefficient between water and octanol (K_{ow})

This gives an indication of relative solubility of a chemical in water and in octanol. Chemicals that tend to dissolve in octanol (high K_{ow}) and not mix with water are said to be hydrophobic or 'water disliking'. Substances that dissolve in water (low K_{ow}) are described as hydrophilic or 'water liking'. Hydrophobic chemicals tend to bind onto organic matter in the environment, including soil, sediment, and the fatty regions of animals and plants (Mackay et al., 1996a).

Hydrophobic chemicals tend to accumulate in fatty tissue in the body and remain in the body for prolonged periods, increasing exposure. They also tend to bioaccumulate and cross the blood-brain barrier (Banks, 2009). Certain hydrophobic chemicals may permeate plastic pipes leading to drinking water supply contamination (EPA, 2002).

Environmental decontamination

Chemicals that are hydrophobic tend to be more difficult to remediate and cannot be decontaminated with water alone (Wyke-Sanders et al., 2012).

Organic carbon-water partition coefficient (soil sorption)

The soil sorption organic carbon-water coefficient (K_{oc}) is the ratio between the concentration of a compound per unit mass of carbon relative to the concentration in water. Chemicals with a high K_{oc} tend to adsorb and become tightly bound to material in soil; they are likely to remain close to the surface of soil and present an ingestion hazard. A low K_{oc} is usually associated with organic chemicals that are mobile in soil (Mackay et al., 1996a).

Environmental decontamination

Chemicals with a high K_{oc} are likely to remain close to the soil surface and can be removed effectively by topsoil removal, also known as 'dig and dump' (Wyke-Sanders et al., 2012).

Persistence (half-life in soil, air, water)

The persistence refers to the time a chemical is expected to remain in the environment. This is often expressed as a half-life (T½) and is the time taken for half the compound to disappear from the relevant medium (soil, air, or water). Most organic compounds degrade in the environment but it is an extremely complex process depending on the properties of the chemical and the nature of the environment it is released to. Factors such as microbial degradation, organic matter present in soil, exposure to sunlight, and other environmental factors such as temperature or pH influence the half-life of a chemical (Mackay et al., 1996b).

Highly persistent chemicals will remain in the environment and result in exposure to the public via skin contact, inhalation, or ingestion. Chemicals such as perfluorooctane sulfonic acid (PFOS) and its derivatives, which are resistant to breakdown in the environment, may also be resistant to breakdown in the body once absorbed and exert a prolonged toxic effect and/or bioaccumulate (Bull, 2009).

Environmental decontamination

Chemicals that do not persist in the environment may not require any specific remediation techniques. Persistent chemicals such as dioxins that do not degrade in the environment also tend to react less with decontamination solutions (for example bleaches). Physical removal techniques such as scrubbing, sand blasting, or topsoil removal may be more appropriate for such chemicals (Wyke-Sanders et al., 2012).

Specific gravity

Specific gravity is the ratio of a density of a liquid or solid compared to a reference. Water is chosen as a common reference media for specific gravity and is given the value of 1. Insoluble chemicals with a lower density than water, such as kerosene, will float on water and are more likely to present a hazard to recreational water users such as swimmers or fishermen. Chemicals that are insoluble and heavier than water (for example mercury) will sink through the water column under the action of gravity until they reach an impermeable barrier such as a sea or river bed (Mackay et al., 1996a).

Environmental decontamination

Oily chemical substances can be contained using booms that float on water to limit the further spread of contamination (Wyke-Sanders et al., 2012).

Chemical partitioning

There is no universal method for predicting the fate and behaviour of all chemicals in the environment, as models developed to predict the behaviour of a specific group of substances may not accurately predict the behaviour of other groups of compounds. However, it is possible to classify chemicals into broad groups that are likely to behave in a similar manner. Mackay et al. (1996b) have proposed a classification scheme that uses the partitioning properties of the substances, as these are key parameters that control their fate and behaviour in different environmental compartments. On a basic level, a chemical may behave in one or more of the following ways in the environment: it can stay in the pure phase of the substance; preferentially partition to the atmospheric environment; preferentially partition to the water environment; or preferentially partition to the solid phases by attaching to a surface or formation of a solid within a solution. Alternatively, a chemical may preferentially partition to organic biological media such as fatty tissue by absorbing into lipids. These behaviours allow the broad classification of chemicals into the categories illustrated in Table 2.2.

Table 2.2 Chemical partitioning categories

Type	Description	Example
1	Chemical partitions to all phases: water, air, and solid	Chlorobenzene
2	Chemical does not partition to air (i.e. vapour pressure $<10^{-7}$ Pa)	Lead, linear alkylbenzene, sulfonates
3	Highly insoluble, hydrophobic chemicals that do not partition to water (i.e. solubility $<10^{-6}$ g/m^3)	Long-chain hydrocarbons, silicones and polymers
4	Chemical does not partition to air or water (i.e. vapour pressure $<10^{-7}$ Pa and solubility $<10^{-6}$ g/m^3)	Large molecular weight substances, polymers (e.g. polyethylene), many elemental metals, and inorganic substances such as minerals
5	May exist as several different species; more difficult to determine fate of compound	Mercury

Adapted from Mackay et al., Assessing the fate of new and existing chemicals: A five-stage process, *Environmental Toxicology and Chemistry*, Volume 15, Issue 9, pp. 1618–1626, Copyright © 1996 SETAC, with permission from John Wiley & Sons, Inc. All Rights Reserved.

It should be noted that this classification is useful for organic chemicals. However, for inorganic chemicals and metals, the environmental behaviour may be more difficult to predict. Toxicity is often dependent on the speciation (particular form) of the compound and this will be influenced by factors such as soil type, pH, and availability of oxygen within the environment (IEH, 2004) (Case Study 2.1).

Case Study 2.1: Waste fire

In the early hours of 1 July 2010, a fire was reported at a waste storage facility. Reports indicated that the fire involved quantities of waste material, including liquid petroleum gas (LPG), alcohols, solvents, paints, dyes, and batteries. Due to the nature of the facility, it was difficult to establish exactly what chemical substances and quantities were involved in the fire. As a result of a breach in the site's bunding (containment barrier), fire-water run-off entered a local watercourse. Following the fire, it became apparent that fire-water, mixed with chemicals, had formed a sludge that had leaked into the ground and sub-floor space of a nearby mail sorting office and residential properties. Evacuated residents had not returned to their homes and the local authority's Environmental Health Officer reported strong fumes when undertaking sampling of the sludge. Table 2.3 explains how the most important physicochemical properties are used to group chemicals, using a volatile organic compound (VOC) as an example of one of the chemicals stored on site.

Initial monitoring revealed that the sludge was contaminated with a wide range of chemicals including lead, cadmium, silver, nickel, tetrachloroethylene, styrene, xylene, toluene, white spirit, dichloromethane, and ethyl acetate. The primary concerns for environmental public health responders were associated with the VOCs such as tetrachloroethylene and their potential to cause irritant effects when inhaled. If released to the environment, there is the potential for vapours to accumulate within confined spaces such as the sub-floor spaces and pose a risk of exposure to inhabitants. There is also a risk of explosion. Tetrachloroethylene has a high K_{ow}, indicating that it has the potential to permeate plastic water service pipes and

Table 2.3 Waste fire incident: Interpretation of physicochemical properties

Property	Tetrachloroethylene (example VOC) Molecular formula: C_2Cl_4	Interpretation
Physical form	Liquid at room temperature	Would usually present a contact (dermal) hazard as a liquid but given the vapour pressure (see vapour pressure entry) it may also pose an inhalational hazard.
Molecular weight (MW)	165.83 g/mole	The molecular weight is expressed in grams per mole. For this substance, the MW is low so this, combined with hydrophobicity, indicates that tetrachloroethylene is a potential neurotoxin.
Vapour pressure (VP)	1900 pascals at 20°C	The vapour pressure is above 1.3 pascals so it will volatilise. This could pose an inhalational hazard and potentially create a flammable atmosphere, especially indoors.
Vapour density	5.83	The vapour pressure (see vapour pressure entry) indicates that tetrachloroethylene will volatilise but the vapour density is above 1.29 so any vapour evolved from the liquid could actually accumulate in low lying areas such as basements, increasing the likelihood of public exposure. The vapour density also indicates that contamination may be dispersed via ventilation of indoor areas.
Water solubility	150 mg/l	The solubility indicates that it is partially soluble in water. Water-based solutions may be effective for environmental decontamination.
Partition coefficient between water and octanol	2500	The high K_{ow} (>1000) indicates that tetrachloroethylene is hydrophobic. Therefore, it is likely to be deposited in fatty tissue and cause toxicity following exposure. The K_{ow} also indicates that it has the potential to be absorbed across the skin or through certain plastic pipes.
Persistence (half-life)	Air: 96 days Water: 98 to 180 days Soil: 510 days	Tetrachloroethylene is highly persistent in the environment. This indicates that environmental decontamination is necessary.
Soil sorption	158 to 501	The low K_{oc} (<1000) indicates it would not be expected to adsorb to solid matter and be mobile in soil.

Source: Physicochemical properties values from the Agency for Toxic Substances and Disease Registry, *Toxicological Profile for Tetrachloroethylene*, 1997, available from: http://www.atsdr.cdc.gov/toxprofiles/tp18.pdf.

contaminate drinking water supplies. If water contaminated with tetrachloroethylene is ingested, its high K_{ow} also indicates that it may partition into fatty tissue and result in exposure over a prolonged period.

The other substances present also had low odour thresholds; this could lead to nuisance complaints. In this scenario, indoor air quality monitoring had not been undertaken, leading to a conservative risk assessment for the properties affected. It was advised that residents be evacuated from their properties until remedial action had been undertaken to remove the sludge, and that indoor air quality and drinking water quality be monitored before re-occupation.

It took seven days following the incident for clean-up of the remaining properties to be completed. Environmental decontamination involving hosing down with water aided removal of partially water soluble chemicals such as tetrachloroethylene. Venting of sub-floor spaces was necessary to remove chemicals with high vapour densities that had accumulated in underground spaces. Sludge was physically removed and environmental monitoring was undertaken to confirm clean-up had been effective.

Summary

In the initial stages following a chemical incident there may be limited information available, such as the quantity of chemical released or adequate monitoring data, to assess the potential impact on the environment and public health. This chapter has highlighted that understanding physicochemical properties is an important skill needed for environmental public health responders to assist in the risk assessment process. Physicochemical properties can influence the environmental behaviour, toxicity, and public health impact of the chemical release and subsequently the implementation of an environmental decontamination strategy. In addition, this chapter has provided a worked example and reference tables to introduce the practical importance of the interpretation of physicochemical properties to the lay reader.

References

Agency for Toxic Substances and Disease Registry (1997). *Toxicological Profile for Tetrachloroethylene*. Available at: http://www.atsdr.cdc.gov/substances/toxsubstance.asp?toxid=48 [Accessed April 2013].

Banks, A. (2009). Characteristics of compounds that cross the blood-brain barrier. *BMC Neurology*, **9** (Suppl 1):S3.

Bull, S. (2009). *Perfluorooctane Sulfonate (PFOS) and Perfluorooctanoic Acid (PFOA)*. Health Protection Agency: Compendium of Chemical Hazards. Available at: http://www.hpa.org.uk/webc/HPAwebFile/HPAweb_C/1246260032570 [Accessed March 2013].

Chemical Abstract Service (2013). *CAS Registry 2013*. Available at: http://www.cas.org/expertise/cascontent/registry/index.html [Accessed March 2013].

Dahl, A. R. (1990). Contemporary issues in toxicology. Dose concepts for inhaled vapors and gases. *Toxicology and Applied Pharmacology*, **103**:2, 185–197.

Department of the Environment, Transport and the Regions (1999). *Environmental Sampling After a Chemical Accident*. The Stationery Office, London.

Environmental Protection Agency (2002). *Permeation and Leaching. Office of Ground Water and Drinking Water Distribution System Issue Paper*. Available at: http://water.epa.gov/lawsregs/rulesregs/sdwa/tcr/upload/permeationandleaching.pdf [Accessed April 2013].

Institute for the Environment and Health (2004). *A Screening Method for Ranking Chemicals by their Fate and Behaviour in the Environment and Potential Toxic Effects in Humans Following*

Non-occupational Exposure. (Web Report W14). Available at http://www.cranfield.ac.uk/about/people-and-resources/schools-and-departments/school-of-applied-sciences/groups-institutes-and-centres/ieh-reports-/human-exposure-and-risk-assessment/w14.pdf [Accessed March 2013].

Mackay, D., Di Guardo, A., Paterson, S., and Cowan C. E. (1996a). Evaluating the environmental fate of a variety of types of chemicals using the EQC model. *Environmental Toxicology and Chemistry*, **15**, 1627–1637.

Mackay, D., Di Guardo, A., Paterson, S., Kicsi, G., and Cowan, C. E. (1996b). Assessing the fate of new and existing chemicals: A five-stage process. *Environmental Toxicology and Chemistry*, **15**, 1618–1626.

Occupational Safety and Health Administration (2002). *Health and Technical Assistance for the World Trade Center (WTC) Dust Cleaning Program OSHA Activity*. Available at: htpps://www.osha.gov/nyc-disaster/wtc-final-residential-dust-cleanup-program.pdf [Accessed April 2013].

Royal Society of Chemistry (2013). *Chemspider. The free chemical database*. Available at: http://www.chemspider.com/ACDLabs.aspx [Accessed April 2013].

Wyke-Sanders, S., Brooke, N., Dobney, A., Baker, D., and Murray, V. (2012). *UK Recovery Handbook for Chemical Incidents*. Health Protection Agency. Available at: http://www.hpa.org.uk/Publications/RemediationAndEnvironmentalDecontamination/1205UKrecoveryhandbookforchemincidents [Accessed April 2013].

Chapter 3

Key concepts and framework for investigation

Camilla Ghiassee, Graham Urquhart, Raquel Duarte-Davidson, Jo Wilding, Charlotte Landeg-Cox, and Allister Gittins

Learning objectives

By the end of this chapter the reader will be able to:
- understand commonly used terms and definitions
- understand general environmental legislation and its relevance to public health
- describe and understand the key principles of risk assessment for public health professionals
- describe basic principles of geographic information systems (GIS) and dispersion models
- describe general principles of environmental sampling and monitoring, including analyses.

Introduction

The following section discusses principal concepts linking environmental science and public health, otherwise referred to as environmental public health. Scientific tools used for assessing the impact of environmental pollutants on health and informing health risk assessments are explained.

The chapter also describes the general regulatory framework for the protection of the environment and health and introduces common terms and definitions and their relevance and application. Many of the topics introduced are dealt with in more detail in the previous and subsequent chapters of the book.

Common terms and definitions in environmental science

Environmental science and environmental health

Environmental science refers to the multi-disciplinary branch of science concerned with the relationships and interactions between biotic and abiotic factors or systems. The synergies and interconnectedness between physical, chemical, and biological elements of the environment are at the core of the discipline. Air, water, land, climate, and bio-geochemical cycles are the key aspects of environmental science that are most pertinent to the human health context of this book.

Environmental health is a term commonly used to define the aspect of environmental science that influences the environmental determinants of (human) health. The World Health Organization (WHO, 2013) defines 'environmental health' as:

> 'all the physical, chemical, and biological factors external to a person . . . It encompasses the assessment and control of those environmental factors that can potentially affect health. This definition excludes behaviour not related to environment, as well as behaviour related to the social and cultural environment, and genetics.'

Environmental health has become more prominent in political and regulatory agendas, as globalisation, population growth, and associated human activities have changed the state of the natural environments. Environmental public health is a subset of environmental health as it focusses on the interaction between the external environment and health. However, it is narrower in its scope, covering the environmental compartments of air, water, and land and addressing chemical, radiation, and noise hazards affecting human health.

Sources of pollution

Pollution sources can be described as point or non-point sources:

- **Point sources** refer to discrete, localised, and discernible discharges of contaminants into the environment (for example emissions from incinerator chimney stacks). In most instances the emission source is identifiable and can often be measured and controlled.
- **Non-point sources** may be referred to as diffuse or fugitive sources, and are releases of contaminants into the environment from multiple sources that are difficult to distinguish and quantify (for example run-off from fertilisers and manure spread on land entering watercourses).

Contamination can result from either natural or anthropogenic (man-made) activities. An example of a natural source of pollutants is the release of gases and particulate matter during a volcanic eruption. Common anthropogenic sources are emissions from vehicles and shipping.

Understanding the composition of the pollutants is especially important for informing the environmental management or remediation options. In the case of air quality, contaminants and pollutants are often referred to as either primary or secondary. A primary pollutant will be one that is directly emitted into the atmosphere by virtue of the natural or anthropogenic activity that results in its release. Secondary pollutants are those that, after being emitted, undergo physicochemical transformations, mostly due to photochemical reactions in the atmosphere. Examples of primary and secondary pollutants are:

- primary pollutants emitted directly into the air from car exhausts, for example carbon monoxide (CO) and nitric oxide (NO)
- secondary pollutants produced via transformation after emission from a car exhaust, for example ground level ozone (O_3).

Some pollutants fall into both categories, for example nitrogen dioxide (NO_2) can be emitted directly from vehicle exhausts and is also formed in the atmosphere when nitric oxide (NO) is released from the exhaust fumes and reacts with hydroxyl radicals in the atmosphere (see Chapter 4).

Air, water, and land all have background (or baseline) levels of chemicals that must be considered when quantitative assessments are required for investigations. In the UK, the Environment Agency's Soil and Herbage Pollutant Survey 2007 (Environment Agency, 2007) assessed the concentrations of a variety of chemical pollutants including dioxins, polycyclic aromatic hydrocarbons (PAHs), and metals in surface soils and herbage. The results provide a reliable baseline of concentrations of those pollutants in the UK and show significant differences between urban, rural, and industrial soils and herbage. For most of the trace elements analysed, urban and industrial soils are said to have, on average, three times the concentrations of rural 'background' soils and herbage.

The presence of a chemical in the environment does not always lead to exposure or adverse health effects; however, the way in which a chemical might be described in the environment (for example chemical contamination) can be important. For example, the contaminated land regime in the UK, based upon the Environmental Protection Act of 1990, specifies that land must fulfil the SPOSH (significant possibility of significant harm) criteria in relation to human or ecological health for it to be labelled 'contaminated'. Chapter 6 discusses contaminated land risk assessment and legislation in more detail, but this point highlights the political nature of the words environmental public health professionals use to describe environmental media that have been affected by anthropogenic activity.

Sensitive receptors

In terms of environmental public health, sensitive receptors are people who may be affected by lower levels of exposure due to their age (i.e. the very young or elderly), habits (for example hand to mouth behaviour increasing their exposure to pollutants through ingestion, or high intake of home grown produce), or health condition (for example immunosuppressed, asthmatic, heart conditions). Sensitive receptors include, but are not limited to, people in hospitals, schools, day care facilities, housing for the elderly, and convalescent facilities. Sensitive receptors are sometimes referred to as vulnerable receptors.

Environment legislation

Brief history of environmental protection legislation in England and Wales

In England and Wales, environmental controls can be traced back to medieval statutes based on small-scale pollution and the development of private law principles to deal with threats to communal assets such as water. The first anti-pollution act, primarily concerned with unhygienic nuisances, was passed in 1388 by the English Parliament, forbidding the throwing of rubbish into ditches, rivers, and other waters. However, the main focus was on the protection of private and common property, rather than the 'environment' itself. The Industrial Revolution (1760–1840) led to the development of public controls specifically related to environmental protection in the UK. Legislative provisions were developed in response to public health problems in the mid-nineteenth century, commencing with the Public Health Act 1848 (Calman, 1998) and culminating in the landmark Public Health Act 1875. The local boards of health established under the Public Health Act 1848 had authority to deal with poverty, housing, water supplies, sewerage, the environment, removal of waste, and quality of foods. The aim of the public health acts was a move to a more proactive approach in controlling public health and environmental quality.

The Public Health Act 1936 consolidated previous public health legislation, which was further consolidated and updated in the Environmental Protection Act 1990. The term 'environmental protection' is used to encompass the environment and human health.

During the 1990s, UK environmental legislation was consolidated within a smaller number of acts:

- **Environmental Protection Act 1990** (as amended) introduced the first integrated system of pollution control, which took into account the potential impact on all three environmental media (land, air, and water) with regards to the most polluting industrial processes and set emission limits and discharge consents. Its purpose was to prevent the transfer of pollution from one environmental medium to another. The act is divided into several parts, including legislation for Integrated Pollution Control (IPC) and Air Pollution Control by Local Authorities (Part I), Waste on land (Part II), Contaminated land (Part IIA), and Statutory Nuisances and Clean Air (Part III). Part I is enforced by the Environment Agency and Parts II and III are enforced by local authorities.

- **Water Resources Act 1991** (as amended by the Water Act 2003) consolidated legislation on water quality and pollution, and water resource management, abstraction, and impounding (such as dams, dikes, and levees).

- **Water Industry Act 1991** (as amended by the Water Industry Act 1999 and the Water Act 2003) consolidated legislation relating to drinking water quality and supply, and waste water disposal.

- **Environment Act 1995** introduced new legal provisions in relation to the identification and remediation of contaminated land and the creation of three regulatory agencies for the UK. It also gave responsibilities to local authorities to manage local ambient air quality.

- **Pollution Prevention and Control Act 1999** implemented the EU Directive on Integrated Pollution Prevention and Control (96/61/EC) and amended it in 2008. The directives cover the control of emissions from specified industrial activities. In December 2010, the Directive on Industrial Emissions (2010/75/EU) was published, which amalgamated the previous seven directives. The Environmental Permitting Regulations 2010, made under this act, have subsequently been amended to incorporate the requirements of the Directive on Industrial Emissions into the Environmental Permitting (England and Wales) (Amendment) Regulations 2013.

European legislation

In recent years the EU and its predecessor, the European Community (EC), have had a considerable influence on the development of environmental legislation in member states. Primary EU legislation is comprised of Treaties, which frame the policies of the EU. Secondary legislation comprises Regulations and Directives. Regulations (for example Registration, Evaluation, Authorisation and Restriction of Chemicals (REACH) Regulation No 1907/2006) become immediately enforceable as law in member states, overriding national legislation. Box 3.1 outlines the REACH regulation and its importance to environmental public health.

The European Commission is comprised of 27 Commissioners and represents the interests of the EU as a whole. The Commission oversees and implements EU policies by proposing new laws to Parliament and the Council. The vast majority of European legislation, including that relating to the environment and public health, is adopted jointly by the European Parliament and the Council. The Council is comprised of Heads of State or Government of the 27 member states, together with its President and the President of the Commission; Parliament is made up of 754 elected members, known as Members of the European Parliament (MEPS). The UK has 72 seats.

Box 3.1 Registration, Evaluation, Authorisation and Restriction of Chemical substances and their safe use (REACH)

REACH was implemented in 2007 under EU Regulation (EC) No 1907/2006. The aim of REACH is to improve the protection of human health and the environment by improved and earlier identification of the intrinsic properties of chemical substances. It places the responsibility on industry to manage the risks from chemicals and provide safety information on them. REACH regulations were introduced as a result of the large amounts of chemical substances manufactured and placed on the European market, over many years, with little information on the hazards they pose to human health or the environment. Within REACH, manufacturers now have to produce safety information prior to a chemical being transported or sold in Europe.

Government bodies and regulatory authorities in England and Wales

There are a number of government bodies and regulatory authorities within England and Wales that are involved in enforcing and advising on environmental public health legislation.

Drinking Water Inspectorate

The Drinking Water Inspectorate (DWI) was set up in 1990. It is the independent regulator of drinking water for England and Wales, providing scrutiny of the water undertakers in England and Wales. The purpose of the DWI is to ensure that consumers receive a safe, clean water supply from their water companies (see Chapter 5).

Environment Agency and Natural Resources Wales

The Environment Act 1995 created the Environment Agency (EA) in England and Wales. Natural Resources Wales (NRW) came into being on 1 April 2013 from a merger of the Countryside Council for Wales, Environment Agency Wales, and the Forestry Commission Wales. The Environment Agency is now an England-only body.

The Environment Agency and Natural Resources Wales contribute to sustainable development and have a variety of pollution control functions, including regulation and enforcement of certain industrial processes (alongside local authorities), discharges to controlled waters, and contaminated land (see Chapter 6).

Local authorities

Local authorities are responsible for the control of local air pollution (Local Air Quality Management; see Chapter 4), the regulation and enforcement of certain industrial processes (with the Environment Agency) and contaminated land (see Chapter 6), and the enforcement of statutory nuisance legislation. In April 2013, local authorities took the lead for local public health protection and wellbeing, with Directors of Public Health being appointed within upper tier local authorities.

Public Health England

Public Health England (PHE) was established on 1 April 2013 to:
- protect and improve the nation's health and wellbeing, and tackle health inequalities so that the poorest and most poorly benefit most
- provide a nationwide, integrated public health service, supporting people to make healthier choices
- provide expertise, information, and intelligence to public health teams based in local authorities and the NHS to secure the biggest improvements in the public's health
- provide an integrated health protection service to ensure that everyone is protected from threats to their health from infectious disease and environmental hazards such as radiation, chemicals, and poisons
- be an executive agency of the Department of Health.

Public Health Wales

Public Health Wales (PHW) was established on 1 October 2009 to provide an expert public health resource as part of the NHS in Wales. PHW aims to protect and improve health and wellbeing and reduce inequities in Wales. PHW has a number of statutory functions, which include the requirement to manage and deliver a range of public health, health protection, and healthcare improvements.

Health and Safety Executive

The Health and Safety Executive (HSE) was established in January 1975. It is a national independent regulator for work-related health, safety, and illness and for protecting the public against risks to health or safety resulting from the activities of persons at work. The HSE is the enforcing authority for, amongst others, the Health and Safety at Work Act 1974 (as amended), the Control of Major Accident Hazards Regulations 1999 (as amended), the Control of Substances Hazardous to Health Regulations 2002, and the EU Registration, Evaluation, Authorisation and restriction of Chemicals (REACH) Regulation (No 1907/2006) (see Box 3.1).

Food Standards Agency

The Food Standards Agency (FSA) was established in 2001. It is a non-ministerial government department, accountable to Parliament through health ministers. The FSA is responsible for food safety and food hygiene in the UK. It also works closely with local authorities (LAs) to enforce food safety regulations. Decisions and advice are based on the best evidence available, including commissioned research and advice obtained from independent advisory committees.

Role of public health in the control of non-communicable disease

Many of the existing Public Health (Control of Diseases) Act 1984 provisions were based on nineteenth century social conditions and were developed piecemeal over a long period. In its Ninth Programme of Law Reform, the Law Commission concluded that public health law reform was overdue.

On 15 November 2007, Clauses 119 and 120 of the Health and Social Care Bill were introduced in the House of Commons to insert a new Part 2A into the Public Health Act 1984 and replace it with more modern and flexible provisions to strengthen the response to infectious diseases and contamination by chemicals and radiation. The Bill incorporates Schedule 11, which contains further amendments of this act and other relevant acts, ensuring that an 'all hazards' approach is reflected within this legal framework for health protection, rather than the previous focus on specific notifiable diseases. The Bill also reviews the action that can be taken at international borders in the light of the International Health Regulations 2005.

The NHS guidelines *Public Health: Responsibilities of the National Health Service and the Roles of Others* (DH et al., 1993) point towards all parts of the NHS reviewing their arrangements to ensure that they are able to discharge their responsibilities to maintain and improve the health of the public, including arrangements for dealing with the health aspects of non-communicable environmental hazards. The guidelines go on to clarify the main types of activity that the arrangements for the surveillance and handling of the health aspects of non-communicable environmental hazards need to cover. These are:

- the continuing surveillance of disease, possible causative factors, and influences in the area, to identify and investigate any pattern of disease that is unusual or novel
- as part of that surveillance, considering the possibility of a long-term raised level of disease in a particular area being associated with a point source of continuing pollution or contamination.

Environmental permitting

It was recognised that some industrial activities could harm the environment and human health unless they were controlled. EU Member States introduced a regulatory system to ensure that particular industries take action to achieve 'an integrated approach to pollution control' in order to secure 'a high level of protection for the environment as a whole' when considering both routine and accidental releases. The definition of pollution in the regulatory regime includes releases to air, land, or water that may be harmful to human health.

Environmental Permitting Regulations 2010 (as amended) came into force on 6 April 2010 and consolidated a number of EU environmental directives to provide industry and regulators with a single permitting and compliance system. The regulations cover waste activities, pollution prevention and control, water discharge consents, groundwater authorisations, and radioactive substances regulation.

The Environmental Permitting Regime requires operators to obtain permits for specified activities or register as exempt, and provides for ongoing risk-based compliance assessment by the regulators. High risk facilities are regulated by the Environment Agency and lower risk processes are controlled by local authorities.

The application process for an environmental permit will address any health and environmental risks associated with the regulated facility. For standard permits (called standard rules permits) a generic national risk assessment will be used. For bespoke permits, site specific risk assessments are required.

The regulations require that all appropriate consultees are informed of applications for permits and for substantial changes. This enables members of the public and other interested organisations (such as public health bodies) to provide comments to the regulator. The EA has 'Working Together Agreements' with organisations such as Public Health England, the Health and Safety Executive, the National Parks Authorities, Natural England, Local Authorities Co-ordinators for Regulatory Services (LACORS), and the Food Standards Agency.

The public health consultee may:

- advise on any particular local health problems they consider relevant
- consider the likely impact of releases on human health (both acute and chronic)

- identify priority substances for control, from both routine and potential accidental releases
- comment on any concerns about cumulative pollution from other regulated facilities in the area that might give rise to adverse health effects on the local population.

Control of Major Accident Hazards regulations

The Control of Major Accident Hazards (COMAH) regulations implement the requirements of the Seveso II Directive within Great Britain in 1999 (Northern Ireland produces its own regulations). The COMAH regulations aim to prevent major accidents involving dangerous substances and limit the consequences to people and the environment of any accidents that do occur. Case Study 3.1 describes the background to the development of COMAH regulations. The regulations require every operator to take all measures necessary to prevent accidents and limit their consequences to human health and the environment.

Case Study 3.1: Major accident in Seveso

The Seveso Directive was named after an accident that occurred in a chemical plant near the town of Seveso, in northern Italy, in 1976. A reactor vessel ruptured, causing the release of a toxic vapour cloud comprising by-products of the process including, most notably, the persistent organic pollutant and carcinogen 2,3,7,8-tetracholoro-dibenzo-para-dioxin (TCDD).

The cloud of toxic chemicals contaminated an area of 15 square kilometres where 37,000 people lived. Immediate health effects included skin inflammation, skin lesions, and chloracne. Wild animals were found dead and agriculture was also affected; people were advised not to consume local produce and livestock were slaughtered to prevent dioxin from entering the food chain. The worst contaminated areas were evacuated while the Italian government implemented costly quarantine and decontamination. Extensive studies continue to assess the long-term human health effects from this incident.

Major accidents have the potential to give rise to a wide range of health consequences and may have far-reaching effects, both on populations local to COMAH sites themselves, and those located further afield (particularly in the event of incidents that lead to toxic gas clouds or other airborne pollution). The Health and Safety Executive (HSE) and the Environment Agency (EA) are the joint 'competent authority' (CA) in England and Wales. In Northern Ireland, the CA is the Health and Safety Executive for Northern Ireland and the Northern Ireland Environment Agency, and for Scotland the CA is the Health and Safety Executive (HSE) and the Scottish Environment Protection Agency (SEPA). The role of the CA is to ensure that the regime operates effectively by overseeing and coordinating the regulation of major accident hazards.

The public health organisations that are part of the multi-agency response to major accidents also have a role in planning and preparedness. Top-tier COMAH sites (sites holding inventories of dangerous substances, at or above quantities defined in the regulations) are required to produce, review, revise, and test on and off-site emergency plans. The plans should include adequate arrangements for dealing with the consequences of possible major accidents and containing and controlling incidents so as to minimise effects and limit damage to persons, the environment, and property.

The preparation of off-site emergency plans is part of a multi-agency contingency planning process that involves the 'competent authority' and other key Category 1 and 2 responders under the Civil Contingencies Act 2004, such as the emergency services, local authority, health organisations, EA and HSE. The off-site plan should be put into effect without delay when a major accident at a COMAH site occurs or when an uncontrolled event occurs that could reasonably be expected to lead to a major accident.

Health bodies aim to ensure that the health aspects of incident response are fully considered in the preparation and exercising of emergency plans. Their input can inform proactive risk assessment and exercise scenarios. Local health bodies will hold information about local population and healthcare facilities (for example capacity and likely impacts on infrastructure and services).

Environmental legislation summary

The underlying aim of EU environmental policy is to promote a resource-efficient economy and safeguard people's health (European Union, 2013). In the UK, most environmental legislation has enacted or implemented EU directives and regulations. Although there is a focus on prevention, the responsibility for enforcing environmental legislation is undertaken by various agencies to ensure both the environment and public health are protected.

General concepts of environmental public health risk assessment

Assessing a risk involves an analysis of the consequences and probability that a hazard will result in harm or cause adverse health effects under specific circumstances. Box 3.2 provides some key definitions of environmental risk assessment.

In decision making, low consequence/low probability risks (light grey in Figure 3.1) are typically perceived as acceptable and therefore there is no need to reduce the risks further. On the other hand, high consequence/high probability risks (dark grey in Figure 3.1) are perceived as unacceptable and a strategy is required to reduce the risks to acceptable levels. Other risks (medium grey shading in Figure 3.1) may require a more detailed risk assessment to better understand the features that most contribute to the risks and/or to decide on the most appropriate options for managing/reducing those risks to acceptable levels. Figure 3.1 shows an example of a three by three (3 × 3) risk matrix (high, medium, low); examples of four by four and five by five matrices also exist to deal with a wider range of categories and more complex situations (for example very low, low, moderate, high, and very high). Generally, the 3 × 3 or 5 × 5 matrices are used in preference to other matrices.

Box 3.2 Key definitions in environmental public health risk assessment

Hazard: A situation or chemical, radiological, biological, or physical agent that may lead to harm (impact) or cause adverse health effects.

Risk: The potential consequences of a hazard combined with their likelihoods/probabilities.

Risk assessment: The formal process of evaluating the consequences of a hazard and their likelihoods/probabilities.

Risk management: The process of appraising the options for responding to risk and deciding which to implement.

Stakeholders: Individuals who are interested in, or affected by, an issue or situation.

Uncertainty: Limitations in knowledge about the impacts and the factors that influence them. Uncertainties originate from randomness as well as incomplete knowledge.

Text extracts from *Green Leaves III, Guidelines for Environmental Risk Assessment and Management*, Defra (Department for Environment, Food and Rural Affairs) and Cranfield University, p.6, © Crown Copyright 2011, licensed under the Open Government Licence v1.0, available from https://www.gov.uk/government/uploads/system/uploads/attachment_data/file/69450/pb13670-green-leaves-iii-1111071.pdf.

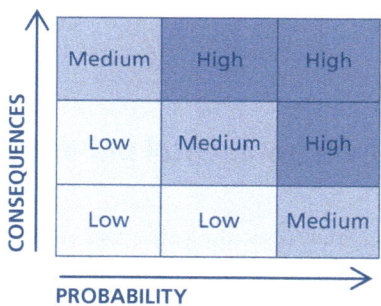

Risk = Probability (likelihood) × Consequence (impact)

Fig. 3.1 An example of a risk screening matrix.

Adapted from *Green Leaves III, Guidelines for Environmental Risk Assessment and Management*, Defra (Department for Environment, Food and Rural Affairs) and Cranfield University, Figure 1, p.7, © Crown Copyright 2011, licensed under the Open Government Licence v1.0, available from https://www.gov.uk/government/uploads/system/uploads/attachment_data/file/69450/pb13670-green-leaves-iii-1111071.pdf.

A structured approach to risk assessment and management

Risk assessment and risk management frameworks have been developed by some countries and by different organisations (for example IGHRC, 1999; US Presidential Commission, 1997; WHO, 2010; Green Leaves III, 2011; HM Treasury, 2003). These offer a

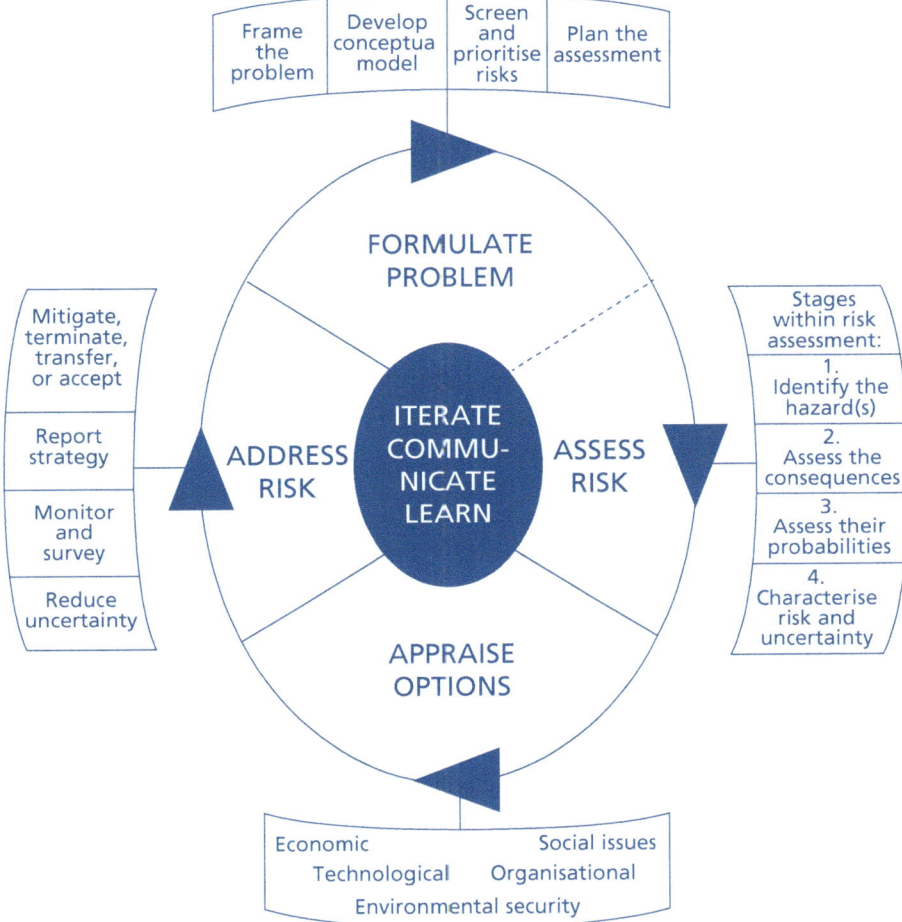

Fig. 3.2 A framework for environmental risk assessment and management.

Reproduced from *Green Leaves III, Guidelines for Environmental Risk Assessment and Management*, Defra (Department for Environment, Food and Rural Affairs) and Cranfield University, Figure 2, p.9, © Crown Copyright 2011, licensed under the Open Government Licence v1.0, available from https://www.gov.uk/government/uploads/system/uploads/attachment_data/file/69450/pb13670-green-leaves-iii-1111071.pdf.

structure to guide decision-makers through the risk management process and help them address all the issues that need to be considered when assessing risks. They also provide relevant information for making decisions on how best to manage those risks. Figure 3.2 shows one example of this structured approach to risk management and identifies four main components:

1. problem formulation
2. conducting an assessment of the risks

3. identifying and appraising the management options available
4. addressing the risk with the chosen risk management strategy.

The framework presented in Figure 3.2 (Green Leaves III, 2011) is based on an earlier version (Green Leaves II, 2000). Green leaves III was updated to:

- incorporate recent advances aimed at improving the potential for stakeholders and the public to become involved in the process
- present recent developments in the tools and techniques used in risk analysis.

The structure shown in Figure 3.2 is a dynamic and cyclical approach whereby risks are reconsidered as new information comes to light (iterative approach) and arrangements are made to implement the lessons identified when assessing the risks to ensure that a preventative approach is followed to risk management. This figure also highlights the importance of effective risk communication and the need to consider social issues; these are key components of the risk assessment and management process and should start early and continue throughout. Emerging risks often generate public concerns because they are viewed as being outside of our control or they are not well understood or not well managed, so ensuring this proactive stakeholder participation helps reduce the number of surprises and secures more beneficial outcomes (Green Leaves III, 2011).

The level of effort put into assessing each risk needs to be proportionate to its complexity as well as to its significance and priority in relation to other risks (Green Leaves III, 2011). The level of effort required will also depend on the ultimate purpose for which the assessment is being carried out, the magnitude of the issue, the resources that can be allocated to addressing the problem, and the time available, costs, and human and technical resource consideration. Stakeholders' perception of the nature of the risks is also a key consideration. The problem formulation stage should help define the extent of the subsequent analysis required.

Problem formulation

Clear problem formulation ensures that the assessment is focussed and that the output from the assessment is relevant, thereby resulting in effective risk management. It also assists in understanding the boundaries covered in the assessment, both in terms of the timeline and the spatial scale. Problem formulation involves framing the problem, defining the question and the desired outcomes. Engaging stakeholders will be required at this stage. This includes establishing basic information about the risk, i.e. the risks of what, to whom, where, and when (for example what are the risks to the local population of drinking this water?). Establishing the scope and objectives of the assessment helps with the selection of the appropriate types of assessment methodologies and provides a rationale for the process that needs to be followed, should the risk decision be challenged or audited (see Case Study 3.2).

Conceptual models can be developed to show a schematic representation of the boundaries of the problem being considered by setting out the relationship between hazards, exposures, and environmental features before analysing these in more detail (see Figure 6.2

Case Study 3.2: Human health risk assessment for a site that has high levels of contamination in soil

Problem formulation

A number of random samples were taken from soils collected at a couple of locations in a UK city centre. These were analysed for a number of chemicals and measured concentrations of dioxins and other contaminants were high. Concerns were raised by these elevated levels, which led to a detailed survey of potentially contaminated sites to determine the extent of the contamination and whether local residents may have been exposed to unacceptable levels of pollution. Further measurements conducted on 80 sites showed that it is likely that half of the sites had high levels of dioxins in soils.

A request was made by the local authority to an environmental consultancy to undertake a human health risk assessment to find out whether the concentrations of dioxins at the various sites had, and would, continue to pose a significant risk to human health. Risks were estimated using measured soil concentrations and the current use of the sites (recreational and as allotments for home grown products). Target populations were identified as children who played in the recreational sites and individuals who grew their own vegetables locally, and their families.

The assessment focused on:

- establishing a Steering Group with key stakeholders to monitor the progress, engage in the risk communication process, and consider the results of the human health risk assessment
- reviewing the quality of the measured soil concentration data
- assessing all plausible pollutant linkages relating to human health
- assessing the risk to human health based on the current use of the land in accordance with guidance and best practice
- producing a human health risk assessment report to inform the local authority of the outcome of the risk assessment and the significance of the results, in order to enable the council to look at the options available to them to manage the situation.

Method

A Steering Group was set up to ensure independence and guide the process. This group had representation from public health, the local authority, relevant agencies (e.g. environment, food standards), and local residents. It had a role in:

- reviewing the health risk assessment and providing support to the public health authority as requested
- considering the results of the health risk assessment and advising on a public communication strategy
- inviting contributions from interested parties.

A conceptual model was developed for a number of representative sites in the city to include recreational areas and allotments (see Figure 6.2 in Chapter 6 for an example of a conceptual model). Using available information, source–pathway–receptor linkages were established (following a similar process to that shown in Table 3.1). This information was used to identify the main pathways of concern and further site specific risk assessment was undertaken on plausible pathways. All potential pathways were considered (e.g. eating home grown vegetables, soil ingestion) and critical receptors were identified (allotment holders, toddlers).

Appropriate commercial computer packages were used to derive daily intakes, which were estimated for ten of the sites (six allotments, three recreational sites, one control), and to be precautionary in the risk estimates a 'worst-case scenario' was assumed for each site (e.g. maximum soil concentrations; large proportion of vegetables consumed unwashed and produced in allotments; a certain degree of soil ingestion).

A report was produced detailing the findings of the risk assessment. To assess the likelihood of any significant risk to human health arising from the sites investigated, the estimated daily intake of dioxins was compared with the corresponding tolerable daily intakes (TDIs) and the findings reported. For most sites the estimated daily intakes were less than the TDI, though exceedance of the TDI did occur in a limited number of sites. The report provided an explanation of the findings; for example, that exceeding a tolerable daily intake does not necessarily imply that individuals will show any appreciable risk of adverse effects during their lifetime, because the TDI incorporates a set of uncertainty factors and the estimated exposure for this site was conservative (as worst-case scenarios had been used in the assessment).

Limitations and uncertainties associated with the exposure and risk assessment were explored and highlighted. These included a commentary on the overall sampling strategy and the exposure modelling. The assessment can only be described as an indication of the likely risks posed by the contamination, and only through further sampling, analysis, and assessment can the confidence in the risk modelling be increased.

The original question was to find out whether the concentrations of dioxins at the various sites had posed, and would continue to pose, a significant risk to human health. The conclusion was that, based on the assessment of representative sites, it was unlikely there would be any significant actual health effects arising from the contamination. For a small number of sites that were examined (5%), the estimated daily intake appeared to exceed the TDI. This is clearly not the same as saying that effects were likely to occur, since the risk assessment deliberately examined a relatively conservative worst-case scenario (and there were also uncertainty factors built into the underlying TDI value). Every effort should be made to continue to reduce exposure from contaminated soils at sites where any contamination remains. However, it would be sensible to carry out some follow-up work to confirm the level and extent of contamination across the sites where daily intakes exceeded the TDI, and the level of exposure for key pathways (e.g. measuring the concentration of contamination in vegetables).

---

in Chapter 6 for an example). The level of detail provided in a conceptual model can vary significantly depending on the level of complexity being considered (for example single chemical and single receptor versus a number of chemicals from more than one source and multiple receptors). The conceptual model is a graphical representation of the sources (S) of a hazard, the pathway (P) by which the exposure can occur, and the receptor (R) (for example groups of people) that may be adversely affected if exposed to the hazard. Existing or potential linkages between these components of a risk (S-P-R) can be set up in a table format with reference to the conceptual model to summarise those relationships visually (Table 3.1).

It is important to plan how the assessment is to be undertaken, identifying the data required and the most appropriate methods for data collection and synthesis. Risks can be assessed qualitatively and/or quantitatively depending on the requirements of the assessment. The amount of information needed for each step of the risk assessment process may

Table 3.1 An example of S-P-R linkages

Hazard	Source	Pathway	Receptor	S-P-R linkage
Dioxin mixture	Contaminated soil	Soil ingestion	Child	Yes
		Inhalation of dust	Child/adult	Yes

also vary, with some steps requiring more detailed, and others less detailed, information gathering.

Risk screening is a useful process to: (1) identify what should be investigated in more detail, either because they may potentially pose a high risk or because there are significant uncertainties around the risk estimates; (2) rationalise why some risks may not be investigated further; and (3) identify risks for immediate action, without the need for further investigation. Following screening, a list of prioritised risks is normally produced to highlight the risks that are of main concern and require a more detailed assessment. Screening assessments are designed to be precautionary in that, where uncertainty remains about the probability or consequences of the harm, these will be escalated to the next tier of analysis.

Assessing the risks

This is the formal process of evaluating the consequences of a hazard(s) being realised and its probabilities. The estimation of the risks typically involves four stages: identifying the hazards; assessing the potential consequences of the specific hazards; assessing the probabilities of these consequences; and characterising the risk and uncertainties (Figure 3.2). The outputs of this structured process provide a judgement as to the likelihood of the risk occurring and its significance, along with details on how the risk was assessed and where assumptions and uncertainties exist.

A large array of tools and techniques exist, ranging from qualitative (e.g. S-P-R analysis, qualitative event trees) and semi-quantitative (e.g. ranking, scoring systems) to quantitative (quantitative fault tree analysis and quantitative exposure assessments) methods. Qualitative methods are simpler and cost effective but more subjective than quantitative approaches. On the other hand, quantitative methods provide less subjective results but are resource intensive, require substantial data and analysis and/or mathematical modelling, and rely on the selection and manipulation of data. As a consequence, quantitative assessments are only undertaken when a decision cannot be made based on the outputs from the qualitative or semi-quantitative assessments.

The four stages in the risk assessment process are as follows (Green Leaves III, 2011):

1. Hazard identification is the process used to identify the specific hazards and determine whether exposure to the hazards has the potential to cause harm.

2. Assessing the consequences (hazard characterisation) involves a qualitative or quantitative description of the inherent properties of the hazard that have the potential to cause adverse health effects. The consequences of a particular hazard may be actual or potential harm to human health or the wider environment.

3. Assessing the probabilities involves an evaluation of the likelihood that the consequences may be realised. There are three measures:

    a. The probability of the initiating event occurring. Many environmental risks occur following the failure of engineering systems, which may lead, for example, to an accidental release caused by a major plant failure, resulting in a hazardous release to the environment and exposure to the population. An example of this type of failure is that of the Bhopal disaster in India in 1984. This was caused by a gas leak from a storage tank, which led to over half a million people being exposed to methyl isocyanate gas and other chemicals (WHO, 2009). Tools such as fault trees and event tree analysis are used to estimate the probability of these events occurring (an example is provided in Figure 3.3).

b. The probability of exposure to the hazard. This involves the estimation of what happens when a release occurs; for example, when a hazardous agent is released into the environment, it may travel some distance to the receptors. This involves characterising the spatial and temporal distribution from the source of release to the receptor, often using dispersion and exposure models.

c. The probability of the receptor being affected by the hazard. The likelihood of harm depends on a number of factors including the susceptibility and vulnerability of the receptor to the hazard, the potency of the hazard itself, and the amount or extent of exposure. For chemical hazards, this estimate is often simplified in terms of the dose–response relationship, which relates exposure to the expected magnitude of harm by certain receptor types.

Depending on the scope of the risk assessment it may only be necessary to assess one of these three probabilities, or all three may be relevant and may need to be considered.

4 Characterising risk and uncertainty. Risk characterisation brings together all the information from the previous stages to provide a qualitative or quantitative statement about the significance of the risks, along with details on how the risks were assessed and the assumptions and uncertainties made in the assessment. A variety of methods can be used to characterise the risks. A basic approach might involve comparing measured or estimated exposure with standard or guideline values (for example environmental

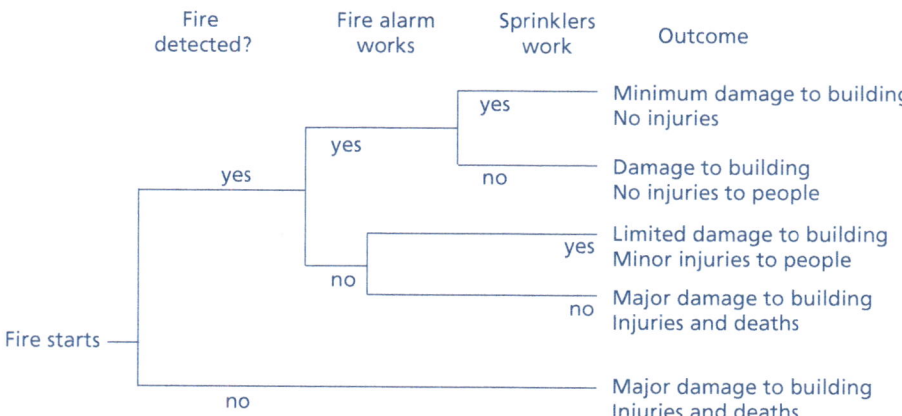

Fig. 3.3 Simple example of an event tree analysis of a fire starting in a building.

quality standards). When using this (or any other) approach, consideration must be given to the uncertainties in the exposure estimates when interpreting the results.

Options appraisal

Unacceptable risks require management to lower them to a tolerable level. Decision-makers need to look at the different risk management options available to, for example, terminate, mitigate, transfer, or tolerate the risks. Options appraisal is the process of identifying and selecting the most appropriate risk management strategy. This process involves looking at various criteria and identifying the best option available, taking into account technical and economic (cost of implementing the options) factors, environmental security (impact on health and sustainability of environmental resources), social issues (e.g. impact on communities), and organisational capabilities (Green Leaves III, 2011). The decision making process can be complex and multi-criteria decision analysis (MCDA) provides a practical way to compare decision options where there are multiple criteria for assessing the options. Based on the selection of the most appropriate option, management measures will have to be put in place to address the risks and monitor the effectiveness of these measures (Linkov et al., 2006).

Risk perception, risk communication, and stakeholder and public participation and engagement

Risk communication has been defined as the process of sharing information and perception about risk. It is a two-way interaction in which experts and stakeholders exchange and negotiate perceptions relating to both scientific and community values and preferences. It includes the promotion of public dialogue between different stakeholders, resolution of conflict and agreement on the need for interventions to prevent the risk. Risk communication should take place throughout the risk assessment and management process as illustrated in Figure 3.2, with the process starting at the problem formulation stage.

Effective risk communication aims to encourage a working relationship that facilitates people's understanding of risk, enables them to make informed choices and decisions as to how best to protect the health of individuals and communities, and promotes their ability to collaborate with agencies in identifying solutions to problems (Cabinet Office, 2002; Green Leaves II, 2000). It requires provision of adequate information that explains the complexities and uncertainties associated with the nature, magnitude, significance, and control of a risk. An important principle for effective risk communication in public health is building, maintaining, and, where necessary, restoring public trust in those responsible for managing and communicating the risks.

Successful risk communication is difficult to achieve and it will frequently be necessary to engage diverse audiences that may hold different values and have different levels of understanding of the messages being conveyed. Provided these complexities are borne in mind, and the objectives are clearly defined, communication can achieve its desired outcome.

It is now well-established that public reactions to risk can differ considerably from judgements that are based on scientific probability estimates and that these differences can be attributed to the complex concepts of risk. Perceived risk is driven by a complex mixture of factors, including individual attitudes and beliefs as well as wider social and cultural values. Risk perceptions may be based on accurate or inaccurate information, and the existence of uncertainties in the evaluation of hazards can also be important. Risk judgements depend on the physical characteristics of the hazard itself and are also determined by broader psychological and sociological considerations. A number of factors may cause anxiety about risks and understanding these can help the decision-maker to identify (in advance) the types of risks that are likely to cause concern.

Research suggests that people tend to be less tolerant of risks that they perceive as being uncontrollable, having catastrophic potential, having fatal consequences, or that bear an inequitable distribution of risks and benefits. This is also true of risks that are unknown, unfamiliar, emerging, delayed in their manifestation of harm, cause irreversible damage, affect certain groups such as children, or affect future generations. Lack of trust and accountability are also factors likely to make a risk less acceptable. Lots of intensive media attention can also increase public anxiety.

Participatory risk assessment approaches have been recognised as valuable methods to support public engagement (Green Leaves III, 2011). They provide a process by which expert and public perspectives can inform each other, allowing a more informed decision and helping to reduce resentment from individuals or groups who feel they are excluded from decisions that directly affect them. The concept of a participatory approach is the engagement of stakeholders early on in the processes of problem formulation, appraising them of the preferred management options and proposing solutions to a particular risk problem. It relies on communication as a two-way process to exchange information and opinions between various institutions, groups, and individuals (Green Leaves II, 2000) and contribute to the development of solutions. However, it requires careful planning, large amounts of time and other resources, and cannot be expected to guarantee the resolution of conflict or controversy.

Key tools for risk assessment

When undertaking investigations, for example, into disease outbreaks, air pollution incidents, or exploring the behaviour and fate of pollutants in the environment, large amounts of information and data can be quickly generated. Recent developments in computing and other technologies such as global positioning systems (GPS), the real time monitoring of air quality, and remote sensing are making the generation, storage, and transmission of data easier than ever. Recently, the use of social media and 'Web Metrics' has allowed the assessment and capture of population opinion and behaviour information on an almost real time basis.

Information typically includes names, addresses, routes, dates, times, and spatial data such as location, height, and topographic and directional information. Often the various data sets would be best used or interpreted in aggregate but this can represent a significant challenge if they are stored in different spreadsheets, databases, or on paper.

For example, consider a chemical release into the environment and the possible public health consequences. Such an investigation will generate a range of data, which may include:

- people who may have been directly or potentially exposed to one or more chemicals
- where they live, work, and visit
- patterns of travel: how, where, and when they travel (vehicle, on foot, route, time)
- possible locations of secondary exposures
- meteorological information including wind direction
- fate and behaviour of the chemical in the environment
- environmental monitoring data.

Once information becomes available, the challenge of how to use it quickly and effectively to help inform risk assessments or communicate decisions becomes evident. This section will consider two tools available to public health professionals that can assist in such processes, these being the geographic information system (GIS) and the dispersion model, and will give examples of how the two can work well together.

Geographic information system (GIS)

GIS is a computer-based information system that captures, analyses, and displays data representing real world situations. GIS enables the data to be displayed spatially, usually as part of a map. It can be very useful to inform risk assessment and risk communication.

A GIS consists of three core parts:

- Data: Information is held in one or more databases, spreadsheets, or tables, which crucially include spatial coordinates allowing the information to be linked to a specific location on a two- or three-dimensional surface.
- Analysis: GIS is interactive, allowing the user to interrogate and analyse the information using statistical and other tools.
- Display: GIS has the ability to display information visually in the form of graphics, maps and tables.

Data

Data stored in and/or accessed through GIS may be varied and complex but crucially must contain a coordinate reference that allows the location to be accurately identified and plotted. Generally a GIS can store data as one of three types:

- Point data: Typically might include address points, case locations, incident locations, and the location of plant or equipment.
- Line data: Information that has a two-dimensional component such as roads, footpaths, rivers, canals, pipelines, power lines, or routes taken.

◆ Polygon data: Shapes with areas, such as property boundaries, administrative boundaries, exclusion zones around incident locations, flood zones, or areas of land contamination.

Any information with a spatial component can be included in a GIS. In the context of environmental public health risk assessment, this information is likely to include locations of sensitive receptors (for example populations within schools, hospitals, care homes, hospices), locations of hazards (for example contaminated land, industrial sites, acute incident locations), and demographic and administrative information (for example population and census data, administrative boundaries). Figure 3.4 demonstrates how point, line and polygon layers can be used to relate possible contaminative historic land uses to current building footprints.

Typically each data set within the GIS is generated as a separate 'layer', which can be overlaid, ordered, and switched on or off as required in the visual display. For persons not familiar with the use of layers it may be useful to imagine that each type of data is plotted on a separate sheet of paper. One can then choose in which order the paper will be stacked, and insert or remove sheets of paper at will. By ordering layers correctly and adjusting the transparency appropriately, it is possible to combine the various sets of data in such a way that they can be viewed collectively. The GIS software allows the user to move around the mapped data and to zoom in and out to view different extents.

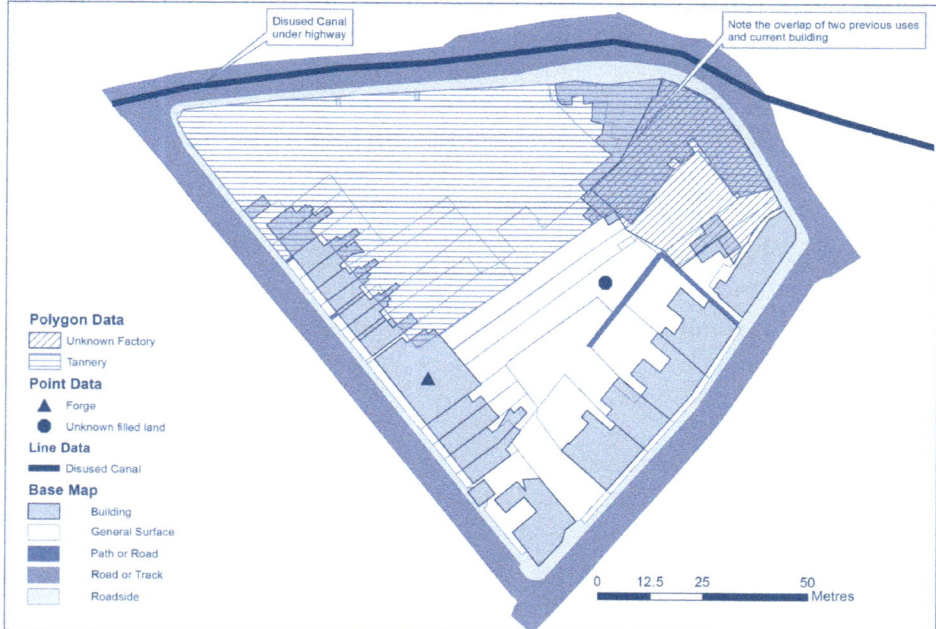

Fig. 3.4 Example of point, line, and polygon layers.

Reproduced from Ordnance Survey map © Crown copyright and database right 2013 with the kind permission of the Ordnance Survey.

Once the data and maps have been plotted, ordered, styled, and zoomed to an appropriate level, the GIS allows for the map to be printed off or exported in a range of graphical formats including jpg and pdf. This allows the resulting plots to be easily shared and incorporated into other documents.

Basic GIS tools

GIS provides a number of ways for captured information to be processed and displayed. There is a range of simple but powerful tools that allows the user to analyse, combine, enhance, and visualise the information. These tools can play a powerful role when using environmental, epidemiological, or public health data, as they allow the identification of relationships, patterns, or trends. The output can aid health professionals in questioning and understanding situations, as well as being able to produce and distribute the information in a format that is easy to interpret for both professionals and the general public.

A range of GIS programs are available, both commercial and free. Whilst they all have unique ways of operating, they typically incorporate the following basic tools:

- Display and move around interactive maps using mouse and keyboard to pan and zoom.
- Search and find a location using address, postcode, or coordinates.
- Find information: underlying data may be accessed either by directly searching the stored data tables or by pointing and clicking on an item in a mapped display. For example, clicking on a school symbol may open a window showing information held in the database on the type of school, age and number of pupils, address, and contact details.
- Selection tools enable selection of subsets of data by spatial proximity and/or by specific single or multiple attributes stored in data tables.
- Simple statistics may be performed, for example summing the values of point data within a specific geographic area.

The use of mapping and simple tools to aid decision making can be demonstrated by the following hypothetical example. Imagine a situation where a specific chemical is being released into the environment as a gaseous cloud. The only information available is a grid reference for the release point. With such limited information it is difficult to undertake a public health risk assessment even though the chemical involved is known, as there is no information on the sensitive receptors.

GIS allows the bringing together of the release location with existing topography, population estimates, the location of potential sensitive receptors, estimated plume direction, and the calculation of summary statistics (see Figure 3.5). This combined information allows formulation of a rapid dynamic risk assessment of the number of people who may be under the plume, and aids decision making processes such as the provision of advice to shelter in place or evacuate people at risk.

More complex GIS tools

In addition to the simple tools described above, most modern GIS include a number of pre-defined tools that enable the user to carry out a number of practical and statistical

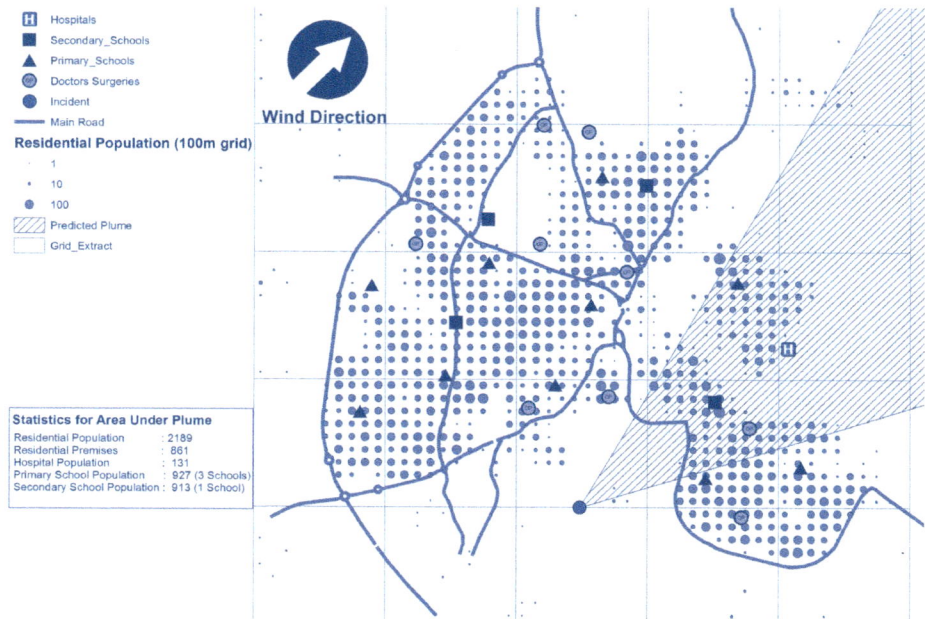

Fig. 3.5 Simple GIS map.
Reproduced from Ordnance Survey map © Crown copyright and database right 2013 with the kind permission of the Ordnance Survey. Population data derived from the Health and Safety Laboratory National Population Database.

actions. The type and number of tools will vary depending on the GIS being used and the licences purchased but some typical examples include:

- Import data: Enables import of multi-dimensional data such as time series data.
- Geocoding: Enables mapping of information in tables where a spatial reference is available, for example grid reference or post code.
- Route analysis: Allows the calculation of best routes based on distance or time.
- Point density: Calculates how many times an event or incident occurs in a specified unit of area. This can be useful when comparing incidence, prevalence, or sampling frequency.
- Identification of clusters, and hot spots, cold spots, and outliers in data.
- Spatial statistics such as interpolation of unknown values using Kriging and regression methods to estimate the relationship between variables in space and identify hot spots and cold spots.

Types of mapping

Typically, GIS is used to produce thematic maps, which have a particular focus on a specific theme or subject. Information is displayed to enable the identification of patterns or trends, to visualise spatial relationships, and to facilitate better decision making. There are a number of thematic map types, and examples frequently used in public health include:

- Simple thematic map: A map where a range of colours or symbols represent spatial location and proximity. Figure 3.5 is an example of a simple thematic map.
- Choropleth mapping: A method of visualising statistical data aggregated over pre-defined areas by shading the region according to the value of a variable in a data table, for example average air pollution concentrations per local authority area, or disease rates per county.
- Dot distribution: A dot can be plotted at a specific point to represent either individual or multiple occurrences of an event at that point. This approach was famously used by Dr John Snow during the London cholera outbreak in 1854, where he manually plotted the location of each death and used the resulting map to help identify the source of the outbreak.
- Proportional symbols: The size or colour of a symbol can be varied to represent the relative size of a variable held in the data set.
- Contour maps: Can be used for data where the changes are smooth and relatively continuous, for example air pollution concentrations around an industrial site.

Benefits of using GIS and thematic mapping

The ability to display information on a map is not new but the ability to easily manipulate and display so much data has only arisen with the advent of modern technology. Capturing the data into GIS allows for the simple identification of spatial relationships such as the position of houses, roads, sources of pollution, incidence of disease, local geography, and administrative boundaries. The visualisation and easy display of multiple layers assists in identifying possible links and relationships to help develop hypotheses and routes of investigation. The information is rapidly produced and can be tailored to make it readily accessible to a wide range of audiences. The ability to clearly show spatial locations and proximity of people, property, and infrastructure helps to inform decisions on emergency planning, public health risks, possible exposure pathways, and health monitoring.

Mathematical modelling

Improvements in measurement can be incorporated into ever increasingly complex models to allow the fate and behaviour of hazards to be studied. There are models to predict how emissions to air will be distributed in the environment, how groundwater will transport pollution, how people will get exposed to soil contaminants, how substances will be transported within the body, and global climate models that consider macro-environmental processes. The role of modelling in environmental science is to predict the concentration of a hazard in different environmental media, which can be compared to environmental quality and health standards.

Mathematical modelling provides a method of predicting outcomes or endpoints on the basis of pre-programmed assumptions, relationships, and formulae, which are combined to create a mathematical representation of a system. Some typical examples where modelling may be used include:

- development control (assessing possible environmental or health impacts from proposed development)
- emergency preparedness and planning
- traffic management
- assessing cumulative impacts of multiple development
- contaminated land risk assessments
- groundwater behaviour and flow
- transport and fate modelling of pollutants released into the environment
- atmospheric dispersion modelling
- flood and tidal risk assessment
- climate and weather models
- predicting the spread of infectious disease.

Models can vary from the relatively simple to very complex but in principle all models consist of three basic elements, these being the identification of available information (input data or source term), the mathematical processing of the information, and finally the presentation of the results in a useable format. Figure 3.6 provides a simplified representation of information that may be included in a typical atmospheric plume dispersion model. The list of source terms, processing considerations, and outputs is not complete, merely representative.

Monitor or model?

When considering public health or environmental impacts it may appear preferable to use actual monitored data made *in situ* over a representative time period. In practice, however, this may not always be practical or possible. In the case of a proposed development, for example, measurements cannot be made as the source does not yet exist, so it may be necessary to predict likely impacts using a model. The same applies when considering the possible impacts of a disaster or emergency chemical release; there would be a delay before monitoring equipment could be mobilised to affected locations and meaningful data gained. For emergency preparedness risk assessment purposes, it may be necessary to consider a wide range of scenarios and combinations of exposures that cannot realistically be created in the real world, so modelling may be used. Even in situations where monitoring is possible, it may be difficult to obtain representative results due to constraints such as cost, available time, hazardous or inaccessible locations, availability of suitable equipment, or the need to provide results quickly.

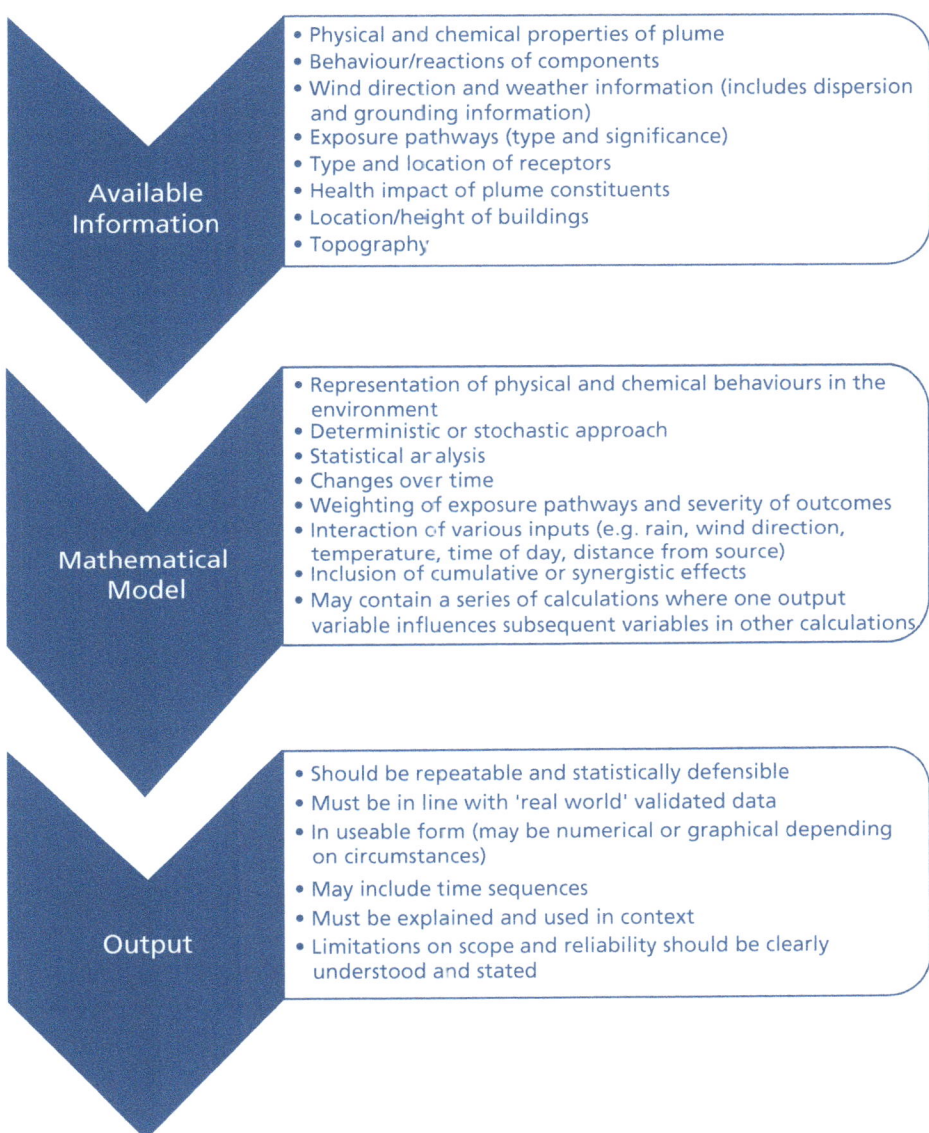

Fig. 3.6 Example of the type of information needed to develop a plume model.

In reality many situations will require a mix of the two approaches. Actual monitoring results may be one of the source terms used to drive the model and at the very least it is useful to have some measured information to validate a model's predictions. The combination of the approaches allows for larger geographic areas to be considered than with sampling alone and for the impact of variations in source terms (for example weather) to be taken into account, whilst at the same time providing confidence that the predictions are likely to be realistic.

Proactive and reactive models

It is useful to consider modelling as falling into two main types. In the case of proposed developments or emergency planning, predictive modelling is used. In the case of acute events such as emergency releases or fires, reactive modelling may be carried out to assist in rapid decision making.

Reactive models Consider the example of a fire at an industrial premises. It is known that the plume released will contain products of combustion (amongst other chemicals) and quick informed decisions need to be made on the likely risk to populations and, for example, the need to evacuate or shelter. In these situations the initial information available is often limited, with the exact composition of the burning materials, the chemical composition and concentration of the plume, and the spread and deposition of the plume being unknown.

Under these circumstances, models can be used to rapidly provide a basic estimation of the likely direction, spread, and dispersal of a plume based on the existing and predicted meteorological conditions. This predicted plume can then be overlaid via GIS to identify where it intersects local populations and to locate any particularly sensitive receptors. The model can be re-run as source term data changes or becomes available, for example a change in the meteorological predictions.

This type of model is 'indicative' rather than specific, but it does provide basic information to allow responders to make information-led decisions that are broadly protective of public health. Additionally, showing the location of roads, rail, schools, and so on assists in logistical decisions such as the location of cordons, evacuation centres, and control centres.

There are a range of free and commercially available models, but as an example in the UK, the Meteorological Office (Met Office) provides this information via a service known as Chemical Meteorology (CHEMET). An example of the typical output is provided in Figure 3.7.

In circumstances where an incident is protracted or where there are specific exposure concerns, more sophisticated models can be run that consider a much wider range of source terms, influxes, interactions, and reactions. These models can be supplemented with measured data from ground, air, or satellite-based sensors. In the case of large or protracted emissions, the spread of the plume can be modelled over time to predict where and when impacts may occur; for example, the spread of radioactivity from the Fukushima reactor, the movement of volcanic ash from the Icelandic eruption, and the plume distribution from the Buncefield Oil Storage Terminal fire (to list a few incidents of this nature).

Proactive use of models In the environment of planning future development, risk management and hazard management models can be a useful tool for identifying possible impacts and consequences during construction, operation, and decommissioning. A wide range of issues can be considered, including impacts on populations, the environment, air, land, and water. Consider the following examples:

KEY TOOLS FOR RISK ASSESSMENT | 47

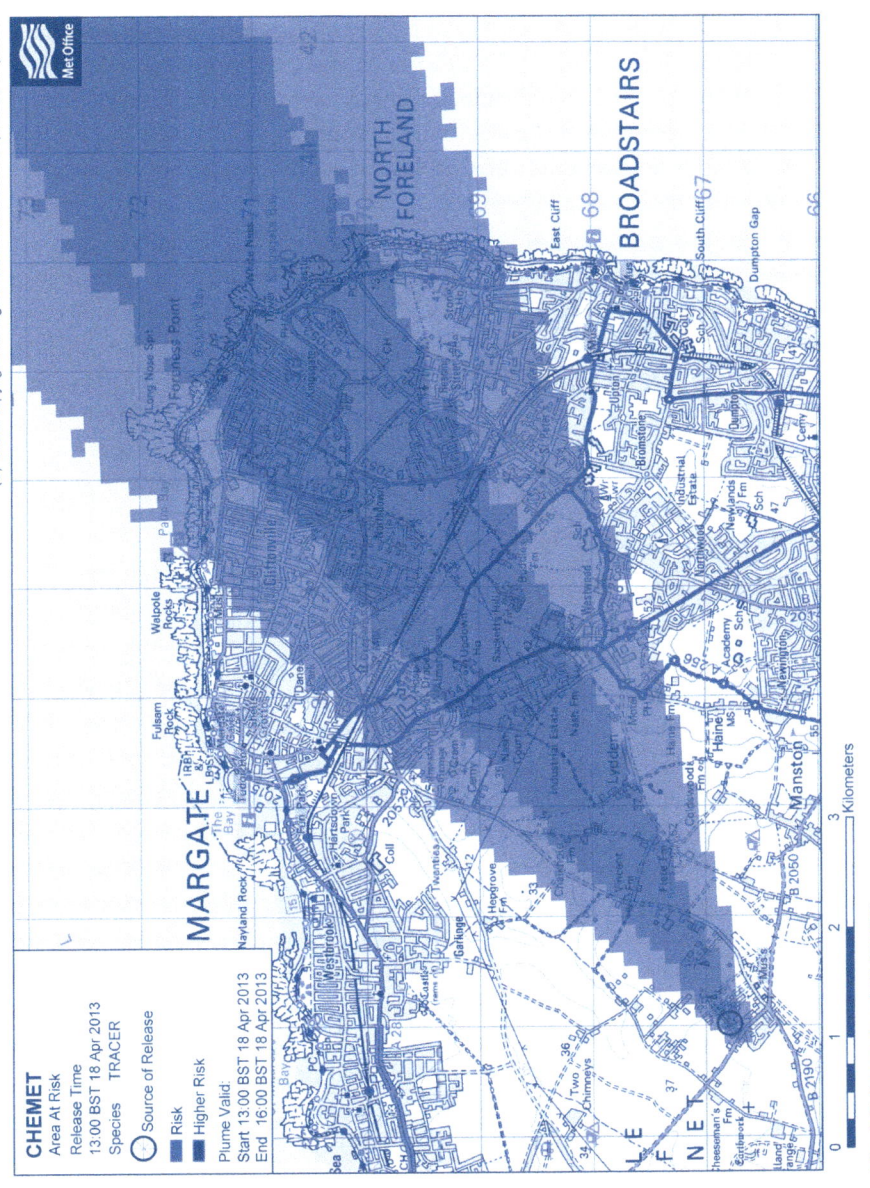

Fig. 3.7 Example of CHEMET.

Map courtesy of the Met Office, licensed under the Open Government Licence v1.0.

- **Emergency preparedness:** A proposed industrial site that uses a range of hazardous chemicals and that falls under the COMAH regulations. Sites in the Higher Tier COMAH category have to include an off-site plan for disaster management and it is necessary to consider both operational and emergency risk assessments. This involves estimating likely emissions, the direction and extent of spread of any release to air, land, or water, local and remote deposition, short-term and long-term exposure pathways, evacuation criteria, and the identification of 'at risk' communities, services, and other receptors. This is a situation that lends itself to modelling. The model can consider a wide range of exposure scenarios, meteorological conditions, and other variables to allow for realistic emergency preparedness.
- **Air quality:** Models are extensively used in the assessment of air quality in the context of existing or proposed pollution sources such as industry, air travel, rail, and roads. The UK uses air quality modelling as part of the procedure for demonstrating compliance with European Union air quality objectives. Background air quality levels have been modelled on a 100 m grid basis for the whole of the UK and these figures are used by local authorities and consultants as the baseline figure when assessing future impacts. Local authorities in the UK have used air quality and traffic models to justify planning decisions and in identification and declaration of air quality management areas. Models are also used to assist in the selection of the most appropriate improvement or mitigation schemes.
- **Traffic management:** Traffic is known to be a major source of UK air pollution and the traffic impacts of commercial, industrial, or housing development are known to be a significant factor influencing local air quality. Traffic movements, flow, and density are typically modelled using a range of commercial products and the predictions of these models are incorporated into subsequent air quality models and assessments.

   Example of GIS use: Arsenic assessment in Cornwall: The geology of Cornwall includes arsenic-containing minerals and the drinking water supply is often extracted from boreholes. Arsenic is a known human carcinogen and consequently the Health Protection Agency undertook a pilot study in an attempt to model the relationship between the known geology and the likely exposure to arsenic. The British Geological Survey was commissioned to produce a simplified geological map that could be used within a GIS system and water samples were taken from a large number of boreholes and water supplies in the pilot area. This information was plotted using GIS to show a relationship between particular strata and the levels found in drinking water. The pilot study has been extended and sampling will now include biological samples from volunteers. All information will be spatially referenced and it is hoped that the combined data will allow the development of a model that will relate the strata from which water is abstracted and actual human exposure levels. If the model can be suitably validated it may be possible to use it to more accurately predict arsenic exposures elsewhere in the UK.
- **Contaminated land:** In order to make some assessment of the possibility of effects on human health, a number of models have been produced by both private companies

and governments. In the UK the Contaminated Land Exposure Assessment (CLEA) software was developed. For further information see Chapter 6.

The advantages of modelling and GIS

Modelling provides a powerful predictive and evaluative tool that helps identify possible public health and environmental impacts from a wide variety of sources. Suitably tested and validated models increase the confidence with which public health professionals may identify at-risk populations, make decisions on evacuation and sheltering, plan for catastrophic events, and identify targets for post-event medical monitoring if necessary.

GIS provides a simple way of bringing together large amounts of information from a variety of sources and integrating it into a single assessment medium. Statistical testing and processing can be carried out within the program and the results directly mapped and displayed. The resulting graphical outputs allow possible linkages or relationships to be identified and the information to be considered with a sense of 'space' and locality. The resulting maps are powerful tools in disseminating information and can be tailored to make them accessible across professional disciplines and by the general public.

Whilst both modelling and GIS are powerful in their own right, the bringing together of the two approaches allows information to be handled, interpreted, and shared at an unprecedented rate. It allows for complex interactions and relationships to be predicted, with the effects visualised and risk assessed in a way that would have previously been largely impossible.

Limitations of use of GIS and modelling for public health risk assessments

Whilst the use of modelling and of GIS provides a powerful way of utilising and presenting data, as with all predictive tools, caution is needed to ensure that information is not being misinterpreted or distorted. There are a number of possible pitfalls that should be considered. These include:

- **Poor data input:** Users of GIS or modelling software must always be aware of the quality, accuracy, and provenance of the base information they are utilising. If information is incorrect, missing, out of date, or used out of context it will lead to incorrect conclusions and results. The accuracy of mapping information is variable and it is possible that similar data sets may contain conflicting information.
- **Uncertainty in models:** Models are a way of predicting events in the real world. They work on the basis of calculation and assumed conditions and behaviours, and include a range of inputs, many of which may be uncertain or include the outputs of another model. For that reason, models should generally be considered as predicting likelihoods not certainties. The uncertainties in any model should be understood and considered.
- **Oversimplification/over-complication:** The output of a GIS may be easy to interpret but there is a danger that the outputs can be oversimplified. It is important that the

map includes the layers necessary to allow information to be interpreted and patterns identified. Oversimplification can result in users not viewing the information in the round and therefore using it out of context. Similarly there can be a temptation to include large amounts of only marginally pertinent information on a map. This makes the output confusing and can lead to misinterpretation.

- **Sample or averaging layers:** The statistical processing of information may provide misleading results in certain circumstances. For example, the simple choice of averaging area can make a significant difference to how a map might display. Consider the following example: when plotting a map showing population density you simply divided the population by the area. However, populations are not evenly distributed, with most people living in urban areas and in certain parts of the country. In the UK, for example, 90 per cent of the population lives in cities, with the largest population being in London and the south-east. The population density (colours on the map) will vary significantly if you choose to map the country as a whole, by regions, by counties, urban versus rural locations, and so on. The possibility that the choice of boundaries and sizes may influence the apparent output must be considered, both when designing maps but also when interpreting information provided by others.

General principles of environmental sampling and monitoring

Environmental sampling and monitoring are important to quantify the potential risks to the public and inform the decision making process. Sampling and monitoring are often referred to as interchangeable but it is important to understand the difference between these terms. Sampling is the physical process of taking a representative sample of the environmental media in question and it can be a one-off process, whereas monitoring more commonly refers to taking regular samples to assess or observe the concentrations of chemicals within a particular environmental medium.

There may be a need to sample and monitor a variety of media depending on the circumstances. For example:

- **Air (indoor and outdoor)**

Sampling of ambient air may be required in the event of a chemical release or fire that could severely impact air quality. This sampling can be used in conjunction with modelling and an appropriate risk assessment to determine whether a given population should shelter in place (for example remaining indoors and closing windows and doors), or temporarily relocate, or be advised to avoid the use of certain areas. Indoor air sampling could also be important, especially if a chemical incident occurred within a confined environment.

Routine monitoring of ambient air is undertaken by most local authorities to ensure that levels of pollutants within a particular area are not likely to cause an impact on health. This monitoring data is used to inform future measures to reduce levels of pollutants (see Chapter 4).

- **Soil and vegetation**

Soil may need to be sampled to assess whether historical activities on a piece of land have resulted in concentrations that may pose a risk to health (see Chapter 6). If the site is used for growing vegetables, for example an allotment, it may be necessary to also take samples of vegetables or other crops grown. Monitoring of soils for gases may also be required. For example, old landfill sites can produce gases that are harmful to health and can pose an explosive risk. Monitoring of these gases may be required on several occasions over a period of time, as they can vary depending on meteorological conditions.

- **Water environments**

If a raw drinking water source or controlled water, such as a river, has been polluted, monitoring will help determine the impact on the wider environment and on drinking water sources that extract from the affected controlled water body (see Chapter 5).

The key steps in undertaking any sampling or monitoring programme are outlined in the following sections.

Planning

Before undertaking any sampling or monitoring, it is important to plan the process. This will ensure that the correct samples are taken to inform the risk assessment and any subsequent decision making.

The planning process contains several key elements:

- sampling strategy
- sampling protocol
- analytical and quality control considerations
- health and safety considerations
- other practical considerations.

Sampling strategy

The sampling strategy is vital to the success of the sampling; it should reflect the key questions that we are trying to answer. A clear understanding of why sampling or monitoring is required and hence what type, quantity, and quality of information is needed should always be established. The sampling strategy should include details of how many samples will be taken, where samples will be taken, at what depths (if sampling soils), and what contaminants will be tested for. This requires a detailed understanding of the site and also an appreciation of how the sampling data will be used in any preceding risk assessment. It is usually advisable to visit a site (if possible) before devising a sampling strategy. Circumstances where this may not be possible are in the event of an acute incident where sampling may be required as a matter of urgency. The location of samples is an important factor in the sampling strategy and consideration needs to be given to ensuring that a sampling pattern is used that will ensure the samples are representative and avoids bias. It is advisable to assign an appropriate number to each sampling location and produce relevant sampling plans (GIS can be used to produce these) prior to sampling in the field. This will avoid confusion during the sampling process and ensure consistency with sample labelling.

The sampling strategy should also include details of what methodology will be used to obtain the sample. For example, it may be that more than one investigation technique is required to obtain the required samples. If soils were being sampled, hand augers might be used to take shallow soil samples but more sophisticated intrusive investigation equipment might be required for deeper soils, such as cable percussive or rotary drilling rigs.

Sampling protocol

Either within the sampling strategy or as a separate document, there should be details of the sampling protocol. This should contain details of how the sample should be taken, consistent with existing best practice or standards. The sample protocol should also advise how the samples should be labelled to ensure consistency between samples and to avoid confusion. The document should also contain details of steps to avoid cross-contamination between samples, for example cleaning of sampling equipment between samples. It should also detail what equipment and sampling container should be used to obtain the sample. The type of sampling container is very important to ensuring sampling integrity. For example, soil and water samples that are being tested for volatile contaminants may need to be stored in an amber jar or vial and filled to the top to prevent loss of volatiles for the analysis. Suitability of sample containers and sample size may be sought from the analytical laboratory(s) that will be conducting the analyses. The sampling protocol should also detail how the samples will be stored and arrangements for analysis. Appropriate storage of samples is also important to sample integrity and this includes factors such as ensuring that the samples are transported in suitable containers and at the right temperature.

Analytical and quality control considerations

In addition to the sampling containers and storage already discussed, there are other important analytical considerations that should be addressed at the planning stage. An initial consideration is selecting a suitable laboratory to undertake the analysis, as not all laboratories are able to undertake certain types of analysis. For specialist analysis there may only be one or two laboratories in the country that can undertake it. Analysis should be carried out by standard methods at an accredited UKAS (UK Accreditation Service) laboratory, at which satisfactory quality assurance procedures are always used (it should be noted that standard methods are not available for all chemicals and that certain competent laboratories may not be accredited to analyse all samples). It is important to decide on the most appropriate analytical technique for the sample. Some analytical techniques or reporting methods may only provide general information, for example, total hydrocarbons or total dissolved solids. To determine the health impact, more specific information may be required on individual chemicals. Also, for some chemicals there may be different species or forms that have different toxicities. For example, hexavalent chromium (VI) is an acute toxin as well as a carcinogen, whereas trivalent chromium (III) is of relatively low toxicity.

It is therefore important to establish which form of the chemical is present in the sample. It is also important to be aware of the limits of detection (LOD) in the analysis method. If the purpose of the sampling or monitoring is to compare sample results with available chemical standards, then the analysis must achieve appropriate LOD (i.e. at least down to the levels of the standards).

It is important to also consider how quality control (QC) will be ensured during the sampling and analysis process. There are a number of methods that can be used to ensure QC:

- Blanks: These are used to determine the contamination of an analytical process, for example instrument blanks monitor cross-contamination between samples. Trip blanks monitor any cross-contamination that may have occurred between samples transported in the same batch. Field blanks monitor any contamination that may have occurred in the field, for example from ambient air.
- Standards: These are used for calibrating instruments or producing calibration graphs. A sufficient number of standards, representative of the minimum and maximum of the range of contaminant concentrations that are required to be measured, should be used.
- Duplicate samples: These are analysed to check preparation or instrument reliability.
- Blind samples: These are standards or samples of known analyte concentration that are sent to the laboratory (without them being informed that it is a blind sample). The blind samples are an internal check of the quality of the system and sample analysis.

Health and safety considerations

The importance of health and safety should not be underestimated. Careful consideration should be given at the planning stage to any personal protective equipment (PPE) that is required for undertaking the sampling/monitoring, for example chemically resistant disposable gloves. In addition, appropriate risk assessments should be undertaken to ensure all hazards during the sampling process have been considered and avoided or mitigated against. It may also be necessary to undertake a Control of Substances Hazardous to Health (COSHH) assessment if preservatives are being used within the sampling process.

Other practical considerations

There are also important practical considerations to take into account when planning sampling or monitoring. For example:

- Environmental impacts: Measures to be put in place to prevent further contamination. For example, if sampling soils, the soil arising should be placed on an impermeable surface or plastic sheeting to prevent contaminating the surface soils.
- Programme: How much time is needed for the sampling and what resources are available.
- Cost/budget: The costs/budget available will often limit the extent of sampling that can be undertaken. It is important to optimise the sampling strategy so that sufficient sampling is undertaken within the costs/budget available.

- Below or above ground services: Consideration should be given to services such as electric, gas, and water. A survey may be required prior to sampling to identify services at a site.
- Access constraints: The ability to access a site may limit the types of sampling methodology used. For example, if access is limited, e.g. back gardens of houses, it may not be possible to get heavy plant such as JCBs onto the site.

Collection of environmental samples

It is important that the sampling part of any environmental sampling/monitoring programme is undertaken by a suitably trained and qualified individual. Provided the planning process has been given careful consideration and adequate preparation has taken place, the collection of samples should occur with relatively few setbacks. However, there are unforeseen circumstances that can occur; for example, contamination may be encountered in areas where it is not expected. There should be sufficient flexibility in the application of the sampling strategy to allow extra samples to be taken where unexpected contamination is encountered.

It is key that the personnel taking the samples adhere to the sampling strategy and protocol to maintain the quality and integrity of the samples. Some of the common mistakes that occur during the sampling process include:

- incorrect labelling of samples so that they cannot be matched to sample location
- not using waterproof paper and pens so that any notes made on site during wet conditions are not legible
- not correctly filling in the chain of custody forms (these are the forms the laboratories use to track what samples you have sent to them and what analysis is required on them)
- incorrect storage of samples, for example, samples are left out in the sun on a hot day and not stored in a cool box.

Analytical results

Following the careful preparation and sampling, analytical results will be received back from the laboratory. One of the key questions is then '*What do these results mean?*' The following chapters in this book discuss some of the important factors to consider when interpreting the results. However, the results may not provide all the answers and it may be necessary to undertake further sampling.

Summary

The presence of hazardous chemicals in the environment does not mean that there will be any impact on health, and the risk of harm occurring will crucially depend upon the substance, form, exposure route, concentration, and duration of exposure. However, where hazards are encountered, environmental public health science can help prevent harm by removing or minimising the linkage between source, pathway, and receptors using the investigative framework, tools, and practices described in this chapter. Furthermore, when undertaking any public health risk assessment, risk perception and risk communication have been highlighted as aspects of environmental public health that cut across all environmental compartments.

Acknowledgement

We gratefully acknowledge the contribution of Alec Dobney, Jeff Russell, Rebecca Gay, and Yolande Macklin for their technical input and expertise for this chapter.

References

Cabinet Office (2002). *Risk: Improving government's capability to handle risk and uncertainty. Summary report*. Cabinet Office, London, UK.

Calman, K. (1998). The 1848 Public Health Act and its relevance to improving public health in England now. *BMJ*, **317:7158**, 317–596. Available at: http://www.bmj.com/content/317/7158/596 [Accessed 22 May 2013].

DH (Department of Health), Department of the Environment, and National Health Service Management Executive (1993). *Public Health: Responsibilities of the National Health Service and the Roles of Others. HSG(93)56*. Department of Health, London.

Environment Agency (2007). *UK Soil and Herbage Pollutant Survey. Report No. 7: Environmental concentrations of heavy metals in UK soil and herbage*. Environment Agency, Bristol.

The European Union (2013). *The European Union Explained: Healthy and sustainable environment for future generations*. Available at: http://europa.eu/pol/env/flipbook/en/files/environment.pdf [Accessed 30/05/2013].

Green Leaves II (2000). *Guidelines for Environmental Risk Assessment and Management*. DETR (Department of Environment, Transport and the Regions) and EA (Environment Agency). The Stationary Office, London.

Green Leaves III (2011). *Guidelines for Environmental Risk Assessment and Management*. Defra (Department for Environment, Food and Rural Affairs) and Cranfield University. Available at: https://www.gov.uk/government/uploads/system/uploads/attachment_data/file/69450/pb13670-green-leaves-iii-1111071.pdf [Accessed 22 May 2013].

HM Treasury (2003). *The Green Book Appraisal and Evaluation in Central Government*. The Stationary Office, London.

IGHRC (Interdepartmental Liaison Group on Health Risks from Chemicals) (1999). *Risk Assessment Approaches used by UK Government for Evaluating Human Health Effects of Chemicals*. Institute for Environment and Health, Leicester, UK.

Linkov, I., Satterstrom, F. K., Kiker, G., et al. (2006). From comparative risk assessment to multi-criteria decision analysis and adaptive management: recent developments and applications. *Environment International*, **32**:8, 1072–1093.

US Presidential Commission (United States Congressional Commission on Risk Assessment and Risk Management) (1997). *The Framework for Environmental Health Risk Management: Final Report–Volume 1*. United States Congressional Commission on Risk Assessment and Risk Management, Washington, DC.

WHO (2009). *WHO Manual: The Public Health Management of Chemicals*. World Health Organization, Geneva.

WHO (2010). *WHO Human Health Risk Assessment Toolkit: Chemical Hazards. IPCS Harmonisation Project Document Number 8*. WHO, Geneva.

WHO (2013). Environmental Health website. Available at: http://www.who.int/topics/environmental_health/en/ [Accessed 2 July 2013].

Further Reading

Academy of Medical Sciences (2007). *Identifying the Environmental Causes of Disease: How should we decide what to believe and when to take action?* Available at: http://www.acmedsci.ac.uk/p99puid115.html [Accessed 11 March 2013].

Barraclough, D. (2007).*UK Soil and Herbage Pollutant Survey: Introduction and Summary.* UKSHS Report No 1, Environment Agency.

Cromley, K. and McLafferty, L. (2011). 2nd ed. *GIS and Public Health.* The Guilford Press, New York.

Everett, P. (2011). The London Earth field survey: collection of samples and data. [Poster] In: *Cities, Catchments and Coasts: Applied geoscience for decision-making in London and the Thames Basin.* London, UK, 13 May 2011. Available at: http://nora.nerc.ac.uk/14270/ [Accessed 20 March 2013].

Gorr, L. and Kurland, S. (2010). GIS Tutorial 1: Basic Workbook. ESEI Press, Swindon.

Health Protection Agency (HPA) (2012). Compendium of Chemical Hazards. Available at: www.hpa.org.uk/Topics/ChemicalsAndPoisons/CompendiumOfChemicalHazards [Accessed 20 March 2013].

Hurst, N. (1998). *Risk Assessment: The human dimension.* The Royal Society of Chemistry, Cambridge.

Miller, V. (2010). How much legislation comes from Europe? House of Commons Research Paper 10/62, 13 October 2010.

NHSE (National Health Service Executive) (1998). Chemical incidents. In: *Planning for Major Incidents: The NHS guidance*, pp. 97–118. HSC 1998/197. NHS Executive, London.

Pollard, S. (2001). Principles, tools and techniques. In: *Risk Assessment for Environmental Professionals.* Pollard, S. and Guy, J. (Eds) The Chartered Institute of Water and Environmental Management, London, UK.

Chapter 4

Air pollution and public health

Adrienne Dunne, Laura Mitchem, Jo Wilding, and Andrew Kibble

Learning objectives

By the end of this chapter the reader will be able to:
- understand how air pollution is assessed and managed in the UK
- understand the main sources of air pollution on both a national/international and local scale, including both primary and secondary sources
- understand the main health effects of the common air pollutants both outdoors and in the home and who is most susceptible to the effects of air pollution
- understand how health based standards and guidelines are derived and how they apply to public health
- understand what people can do to limit their exposure to air pollutants
- understand the role of local authorities and public health in reducing the impacts of air pollution.

Introduction

Indoor and outdoor pollutants that change the natural characteristics of the air we breathe can affect health. When considering air pollution, the focus is often on man-made (or anthropogenic) pollutants, for example, the products of combustion from burning fossil fuels, or emissions from motor vehicles or industry. However, other contributions should be considered, such as those arising from natural sources: pollen, smoke from wildfires, ash from volcanoes, and sand particles from deserts lifted and transported on the wind, to name but a few. The predominance of different sources and pollutants will vary hourly, daily, seasonally, and geographically. There are also many sources of indoor air pollution such as domestic heating, cooking, and second-hand cigarette smoke, which are often forgotten.

Although air pollution has decreased significantly in recent decades, current levels of urban air pollutants in the UK and Europe are still responsible for adverse impacts on health. This chapter will consider key anthropogenic air pollutants, their sources, and their impacts on health, together with measures taken to control them and minimise public exposure.

Legislation

History of air quality legislation in the UK and Europe

We often think of air pollution as a modern day issue; however, it was a problem in London as far back as medieval times, when coal burning was recognised as a contributing factor to poor air quality. Several centuries later, in a bid to convince King Charles II to tackle the air pollution in London, John Evelyn vividly described the invasive 'aer', 'smoak', and heavy smogs that blighted the city. Nevertheless, measures to tackle the problem were piecemeal and largely ineffective.

Air quality legislation today stems from the London Smogs between 1948 and 1962, notably the smog of 1952, resulting from the burning of coal (see Case Study 4.1).

Sources of air pollution have changed considerably since the 1950s and air pollution is now considered to be a local, national, and international (i.e. transboundary) problem. Legislation has adapted accordingly and has shifted its focus from controlling the sources of air pollution to specific pollutants in ambient air.

In 1979, the UK and other European countries, the US, Canada, and Russia signed the United Nations Economic Commission for Europe's (UNECE) Convention on Long-Range Transboundary Air Pollution (CLRTAP). Initially focussed on reducing sulphur dioxide (SO_2) emissions and the exchange of information between members, the Convention has been extended to cover other air pollutants under eight protocols that identify specific measures to be taken to cut emissions of air pollutants. The most prominent protocol to emerge is the Gothenburg Protocol, which was introduced to abate acidification, eutrophication, and ground-level ozone, with the aim of protecting human health and the natural environment. The protocol set national emission limits (tonnes per year) for SO_2, oxides of nitrogen (NO_x), ammonia (NH_3), and volatile organic compounds (VOCs) to be met from 2010 onwards. Additionally, the protocol set tight limit values for specific emission sources (for example combustion plant, electricity production, dry cleaning, and vehicles). Implementation into European law came via the National Emission Ceilings Directive (2001/81/EC), which was subsequently made into UK law as the National Emission Ceilings Regulations 2002. The protocol was amended in 2012 to include national emission reduction commitments to be achieved in 2020 and beyond.

Case Study 4.1: The London smog

The London smog of 1952 is regarded as the worst air pollution event ever recorded in the UK. It was caused by a period of cold weather combined with windless anticyclonic conditions. The weather preceding the smog was very cold and this resulted in people burning a lot of coal to keep their houses heated. Pollution from domestic heating, emissions from a number of coal fired power stations, and other sources such as vehicle emissions combined with fog to form a thick layer of smog that covered the city and lasted from 5–9 December.

The pollution in the smog had a major impact on health. Government reports at the time estimated that 4000 people had died prematurely and a further 10,000 were ill due to the smog. While the number of fatalities directly related to air pollution is unknown, recent re-analysis of health and pollution data from this event suggest that mortality from air pollution during this period could be as high as 12,000.

The event had a significant impact on regulation, research into air pollution, and public awareness of the impact of air pollution on health. The Clean Air Act 1956 (and later the Clean Air Act 1968) was passed in response to this smog, introducing a number of measures to reduce air pollution. Among these was a requirement for cleaner domestic fuels and the creation of smoke control areas in some towns and cities. The act also introduced measures to move power stations away from major cities and increase stack height to aid dispersion of emissions.

The Clean Air Act 1993, which is currently undergoing review, is a consolidation of the 1956 and 1968 Clean Air Acts.

Within Europe, actions to reduce air pollution are taken at a national and European Union level, as well as through international conventions. The first air quality related EU Directive (80/779/EEC on air quality limit values and guide values for SO_2 and suspended particulates) was adopted in 1980. Recommendations from the World Health Organization (WHO) Air Quality Guidelines, originally published in 1987 and revised in 2006, form the basis for values laid out in EU Directives, which also take into account cost and feasibility.

Current UK and EU air quality legislation

Due to the transboundary nature of air quality, UK policy is developed alongside, and in cooperation with, other EU nations. The EU has been working to improve air quality since the 1970s using a variety of measures. These include the control of emissions to the atmosphere, improving fuel quality and vehicle engine standards, and integrating environmental protection into the transport and energy sectors.

The UK air quality standards and objectives are based on the limit values in ambient air set by Directive 1999/30/EC for SO_2, nitrogen dioxide (NO_2), NO_x, particulate matter, and lead. This directive was implemented into UK law through Air Quality Regulations. Separate regulations were introduced for England, Scotland, Wales, and Northern Ireland. The air quality objectives set out in the Air Quality (England) Regulations 2000, as amended by the Air Quality (England) (Amendment) Regulations 2002, provide the statutory basis for air quality in England.

Directive 2008/50/EC on ambient air quality and cleaner air for Europe consolidates most existing EU air quality legislation introduced since 1985 into a single directive (excluding the Fourth Daughter Directive 2004/107/EC relating to arsenic, cadmium, mercury, nickel, and polycyclic aromatic hydrocarbons in ambient air). Directive 2008/50/EC was made law in England through the Air Quality Standards Regulations 2010 (SI 2010 No. 1001), which includes the Fourth Daughter Directive (2004/107/EC).

Policy on how air quality is assessed and managed is based on measures agreed at national and international levels, as described in the Air Quality Strategy for England, Scotland, Wales and Northern Ireland. The first Air Quality Strategy was published in 1997, and reviewed in 2000 and 2007. The current Air Quality Strategy (2007) for England,

Scotland, Wales and Northern Ireland sets out direction for work and planning on air quality issues, the air quality standards and objectives to be achieved, and a policy framework for tackling all regulated pollutants. The aim of the strategy is to improve air quality and protect public health.

Standards and guidelines: development and use

There are a wide range of terms and concepts in national air quality legislation and international directives; for example, standards, objectives, limit values, and target values:

- Standards are the permissible concentrations set for eight air pollutants in the UK. They are based on an assessment of the effects of each pollutant on human health, including the effects on sensitive subgroups or on ecosystems.
- Objectives are standards with an associated target date by which a standard must be achieved. Objectives may include a permitted number of exceedances per year.
- Limit values are used in EU Directives. They are legally binding EU parameters that must not be exceeded. They comprise a concentration value, an averaging time over which it is to be measured, the number of exceedances allowed per year, if any, and a date by which it must be achieved. Limit values may be set for different end points, for example human health or ecosystems.
- Target values are used in some EU Directives, and although they are not legally binding, the intention is that member states should take necessary measures to achieve them whilst not incurring disproportionate costs.
- Guidelines (such as those presented by the WHO) are guidance levels to aid national and local authorities in making risk assessment and risk management decisions when pollutants are present in air. They provide a basis for protecting public health from adverse effects of air pollutants and can be used to eliminate or reduce exposure to those pollutants that are known or likely to be hazardous to human health or wellbeing (WHO, 2000). These are not legally binding.

The air quality objectives for the UK are laid out in the 2007 Air Quality Strategy (see Table 4.1). At a minimum, these are equivalent to the standards set in EU legislation but some are more stringent. Unless an objective in the Strategy is mirrored in EU legislation, there is no legal requirement for it to be met. As of now, all the objectives, with the exception of that for $PM_{2.5}$, should be met. The limit value set for $PM_{2.5}$ should be achieved by 2015.

Local air quality management (LAQM)

The Environment Act 1995 and the Environment (Northern Ireland) Order 2002 introduced the system of local air quality management (LAQM). As certain pollutants are best monitored and managed at a local level, the act placed a statutory duty on local authorities to review current and future air quality in their area against objectives in the Air Quality Strategy.

Table 4.1 National air quality objectives

Pollutant	Objective	
	Concentration	**Measured as**
Benzene	5 μg/m³	annual mean
1,3-Butadiene	2.25 μg/m³	running annual mean
Carbon monoxide	10.0 mg/m³	maximum daily running 8 hour mean
Lead	0.25 μg/m³	annual mean
Nitrogen dioxide	200 μg/m³	1 hour mean; not to be exceeded more than 18 times per year
	40 μg/m³	annual mean
Ozone	100 μg/m³	8 hour mean; not to be exceeded more than 10 times per year
Particles (PM$_{10}$)	50 μg/m³	24 hour mean; not to be exceeded more than 35 times per year
	40 μg/m³	annual mean
Particles (PM$_{2.5}$)	25 μg/m³	annual mean
Polycyclic aromatic hydrocarbons (PAHs)	0.25 ng/m³ (BaP)	annual mean
Sulphur dioxide	350 μg/m³	1 hour mean; not to be exceeded more than 24 times per year
	125 μg/m³	24 hour mean; not to be exceeded more than three times per year
	266 μg/m³	15 minute mean; not to be exceeded more than 35 times per year

Adapted from Department for Environment, Food and Rural Affairs (Defra), *The Air Quality Strategy for England, Scotland, Wales and Northern Ireland (Volume 1)*, Table 2, pp. 21–22, HMSO, © Crown Copyright 2007, licensed under the Open Government Licence v1.0, available from: http://archive.defra.gov.uk/environment/quality/air/airquality/strategy/documents/air-qualitystrategy-vol1.pdf.

LAQM forms a key part in the UK Government's and the Devolved Administrations' strategies to achieve prescribed air quality objectives. Not all of the objectives contained in the Air Quality Strategy are included within LAQM; those excluded are the limit value for PM$_{2.5}$, ozone, and polycyclic aromatic hydrocarbons. Local authorities are not legally required to achieve those national air quality objectives prescribed for LAQM; their statutory duty is to work towards achieving the objectives, despite often having little or no enforcement powers over the sources of air pollutants. Attainment of objectives not prescribed for LAQM remains the responsibility of central government.

The local authority review and assessment process under LAQM consists of annual progress reports, replaced with a more in-depth Updating and Screening Assessment every third year. Local authorities undertake a level of assessment that is commensurate with the risk of an air quality objective being exceeded. Where any objective is unlikely to be met following a Detailed Assessment, local authorities must designate those areas as air quality management areas (AQMAs) and take action, along with other relevant parties, to work towards meeting the objectives. The outcome of this is the publication of an Action Plan setting out the measures the local authority intends to take in pursuit of the objectives. Detailed technical guidance is provided to support the review and assessment process (Defra, 2009).

Most AQMAs are declared to tackle air pollution associated with local road traffic networks; over 90 per cent have been declared for transport-related sources of air pollution. There are currently 475 declared AQMAs for NO_2, PM_{10}, and SO_2. An example of LAQM leading to the declaration of an AQMA, for local air pollution associated with an industrial installation, is given in Case Study 4.2.

Case Study 4.2: Local air quality management

Scunthorpe Integrated Iron and Steelworks, and one other integrated steelworks in Port Talbot, are some of the largest industrial regulated sites in the UK. The steelworks' 2000 acre site encompasses an extensive network of internal road and associated vehicle movements. The site has in the region of 150 emission points and many fugitive sources.

Since 2005, North Lincolnshire Council (NLC) have operated a series of PM_{10} monitors around Scunthorpe town and the steelworks to monitor ambient air quality. Continuing problems have been highlighted by the monitoring, which resulted in the declaration of two AQMAs for breaches and potential breaches of the PM_{10} Daily Mean Objective. Previous air quality assessments had identified the steelworks to be a significant contributor to the PM_{10} burden in and around Scunthorpe, primarily through fugitive emissions. Attributing a specific area of the site or activity as the main source was complicated by the sheer scale of the operations, the number of different companies involved, and a number of contributing factors such as traffic in the town and the possibility of agricultural or sea derived particles.

In 2008 NLC published an Action Plan for the Scunthorpe AQMA containing 37 actions, which was revised in 2012. Seventeen of the original 36 actions remain ongoing. In 2009 the EA initiated a PM_{10} permit review for the entirety of the multi-operational site and ambient PM_{10} concentrations in the surrounding area. This was accompanied by a site-wide review of practices against Best Available Techniques (BAT) and resulted in an action plan for the site to reduce PM_{10} emissions.

In 2011 NLC put in place an Action Plan for the Low Santon AQMA designed to engage all interested parties in reducing the number of PM_{10} daily exceedances within the area. NLC has set up a Local Industry Forum where all operators on the steelworks site work together with the local authority, EA, Health Protection Agency (now part of Public Health England), and others to share best practice across the site to reduce air pollution. The purpose of the forum is to identify key issues, agree measures for reduction of PM_{10}, and formulate a memorandum of understanding between all industrial operators at the site, particularly in respect of issues falling outside the scope of environmental permitting. The updated environmental permit includes a fugitive emissions management plan. NLC has produced guidance for developers on development constraints within the Scunthorpe AQMA. The guidance splits the AQMA into two zones: Zone 1 is not suitable for house building due to air pollution levels from the steelworks; Zone 2 requires air pollution to be assessed on a site by site basis. This has yet to be approved as formal Planning Guidance.

Spatial planning and air quality

Air quality considerations should be balanced against other aims of the planning system, such as economic regeneration and the provision of adequate levels of new housing.

The National Planning Policy Framework (NPPF), published in March 2012, is a streamlining and consolidation of previous planning guidance documents. It sets out the government's planning policies for England and how these are expected to be applied.

One of the aims of the NPPF is to prevent both new and existing development from contributing to or being put at unacceptable risk from, or being adversely affected by, unacceptable levels of air pollution. Planning policies are expected to sustain compliance with, and contribute towards, EU limit values or national air quality objectives, taking into account the presence of AQMAs and the cumulative impacts on air quality from individual sites in local areas. Planning decisions should ensure that any new development in an AQMA is consistent with the Action Plan prepared under LAQM.

Environmental permitting and air quality

Certain industrial processes and activities are regulated for emissions to the environment (land, air, and water) under the Environmental Permitting Regulations 2010 (as amended) and are regulated by the Environment Agency and local authorities ('the Regulators'). The aim is to reduce emissions to the atmosphere and to help maintain and improve air quality. The Regulators are required to have regard to the Air Quality Strategy when exercising their pollution control functions.

Emission limit values (ELVs) contained in permits must be based on the Best Available Techniques (BAT), as defined in Article 1(10) of the IED Directive. Statutory ELVs (for example sulphur content of liquid fuels) are specified in relevant European legislation and the sector specific technical guidance. Reference documents for BAT, termed best available techniques reference documents or BREFs, are published by the EU and are the reference for setting permit conditions.

Where an air quality objective derived from EU legislation can only be met by imposing emission limits on an industrial installation that are more stringent than those associated with the use of BAT, then more stringent emission limits will have to be imposed by the regulator. Where UK standards or objectives are the sole consideration in setting permit conditions, there is no legal obligation upon regulators to set ELVs any more stringent than the emission levels associated with the use of BAT.

Air quality monitoring

Fundamental to the management and control of air pollution is the need for good quality data on levels of air pollutants in ambient air. In 1961, the UK established the world's first coordinated national air pollution monitoring network, called the National Survey. This Network monitored black smoke and SO_2 at around 1200 sites in the UK. Over time, monitoring networks have evolved to focus on new and emerging sources of pollutants and today most monitoring addresses pollutants generated (directly or indirectly) from vehicular emissions, such as NO_2 and fine particulate matter. By 1987, the UK had set up an automatic urban monitoring network, which was later merged with a separate rural monitoring network to form the current Automatic Urban and Rural Network (AURN).

This automatic network includes air quality monitoring stations measuring NO_x, SO_2, ozone, carbon monoxide (CO), and particulate matter (PM_{10} and increasingly $PM_{2.5}$). Most monitored pollutants relate to vehicle emissions. The AURN is the most important and comprehensive automatic national monitoring network in the country and is made up of 103 sites providing real-time data (hourly and daily measurements). Data is uploaded via a modem to the network and is publicly available from the UK-AIR (Air Information Resource) website. Local authorities are responsible for operating and maintaining individual monitoring sites and a number of organisations are involved in the management of the network overall.

In addition to AURN, there are a number of automatic networks in the UK. For example, the Automatic London Network is a subset of 14 sites on the AURN, which also form part of the wider London Air Quality Network (LAQN) run by King's College Environmental Research Group. The UK Automatic Hydrocarbon Network monitors a range of VOCs including benzene and 1,3-butadiene. This consists of five sites, located at Glasgow, Harwell, London Eltham, London Marylebone Road, and Auchencorth Moss.

The UK also has a number of non-automatic networks that measure air pollution. Unlike automatic networks, these monitoring stations measure air pollution less frequently (for example daily, weekly, or monthly). Air pollution samples are collected by diffusion tubes or filters depending on the pollutant under investigation, and samples are then subjected to chemical or gravimetric analysis. Examples of non-automatic networks include the Urban Heavy Metals Network, which measures heavy metals in air near industrial sources and areas of population, and the use of NO_2 diffusion tubes by local authorities around busy roads.

Data from such networks are used to monitor compliance with the EU Directive limit values on air quality and national Air Quality Regulations, characterise spatial variability of air pollution, and consider source attribution (Vardoulakis et al., 2011). The monitoring data gathered over the last 60 years have shown trends such as the dramatic decline in both black smoke and SO_2 concentrations due to the introduction of cleaner fuels and technologies, and successful legislation.

The impact of ambient air on health

Health effect studies

Exposure to various air pollutants is a significant public health issue. The evidence for the impact of air pollution on health comes from a variety of sources, including:
- chamber studies, which involve exposing volunteers to known concentrations of gases for specific periods of time and monitoring physiological response
- knowledge of occupational exposure and resulting health effects
- epidemiological studies, for example time series and cohort studies.

Most epidemiological studies of the effects of air pollution use a time series design, where day-to-day changes in mortality or morbidity (usually within a city or geographically defined population) are related to changes in air pollution exposure. A large population is needed for such a study so that the small impacts and changes in health are picked up. These studies provide evidence of the short-term effects of air pollution.

Cohort studies are used to estimate the effects on health of chronic (long-term) exposure to air pollution. These focus on a specific health outcome (for example mortality), in relation to long-term average pollutant concentrations. Such studies take into account other factors (or confounders) such as smoking, diet, occupational exposures, and so on, which might have an influence on the health outcome. The studies usually compare populations from different geographical locations.

Epidemiological studies have been key in providing evidence of the health effects resulting from exposure to ambient levels of air pollution, highlighting that even low concentrations of air pollutants can damage health. These studies have illustrated the reduction in life expectancy and resultant burden on society, in terms of morbidity and mortality, associated with long-term exposure to ambient levels of air pollution (COMEAP, 2010a).

Susceptible groups

Certain population groups are more susceptible to the effects of air pollution; these include:

- those with pre-existing cardio and respiratory diseases including asthma and chronic obstructive pulmonary disease (COPD)
- the elderly
- the very young.

Short-term exposure to elevated levels of air pollution is known to exacerbate pre-existing conditions and this can result in the need for treatment and increased hospital admissions. Elevated ozone levels have been linked to an increased use of asthma medication. Asthma is a long-term condition affecting the airways of the lungs and is characterised by recurrent attacks of breathlessness, tightness in the chest, coughing, and wheezing. Symptoms may occur several times in a day or week and for some individuals they become worse during physical activity or at night (WHO, 2011). Treatment allows patients to manage their symptoms. Asthma is prevalent in Western society and the UK has one of the highest rates of asthma worldwide, accounting for over 79,000 hospital admissions and approximately 1000 deaths annually, the majority of which are preventable (Department of Health, 2012). The causes of asthma are not well understood and those with the condition have different triggers for symptoms. It is recognised that air pollution can cause an exacerbation of asthma symptoms in those individuals who already suffer from it, and may even play a part in initiating the onset of asthma in some susceptible individuals who live near busy roads, particularly roads carrying high numbers of heavy goods vehicles (COMEAP, 2010b).

Current studies are considering the association between patients with COPD, elevated levels of air pollution, and hospital admissions. COPD is a lung disease characterised by airflow obstruction or limitation. It leads to lung airway damage, causing them to become narrower and making it harder for air to get in and out. It is a progressive disorder; lung damage cannot be reversed but early diagnosis and treatment can help to slow the decline in lung function and lengthen the period in which someone can enjoy an active life (Department of Health, 2012). The prevalence and health burden of COPD is predicted to increase in the coming decade to be one of the leading causes of mortality in the world by 2020 (WHO, 2008). COPD is the second most common cause of emergency hospital admission and one of the most costly in-patient conditions treated by the NHS (Department of Health, 2012).

There is also a growing body of evidence linking air pollution with other health effects. Time series studies have indicated death to be brought forward following exposure to certain air pollutants, for example particulate matter, for susceptible individuals such as those with pre-existing cardiorespiratory disease. Of particular concern are the possible impacts of air pollution on infants and young children due to prenatal and early life exposure, such as low birth weight.

One in five people suffer from respiratory or cardiovascular complaints that can be made worse by air pollution. It is difficult to calculate the cost of the impact of air pollution on society; however, the estimated cost of the health impact of anthropogenic particulate air pollution equals tens of billions of pounds a year. Therefore, improvements in air quality will have both health and economic benefits. There is also a strong link between air pollution and deprivation. Areas with the highest deprivation tend to have the highest levels of air pollution, often as a result of the close proximity to busy roads. Furthermore, deprived communities will also have poorer health than less deprived communities, as higher prevalence of underlying existing diseases will make them more susceptible to the effects of air pollution.

Pollutants, sources, and impact on health

Particulate matter

Particulate matter is a term used to describe particles and liquid droplets suspended in air. In the UK, particulate matter is a complex mix of varying particle size and composition. It can be natural or anthropogenic (for example particulate matter generated from the combustion of fossil fuels). Composition is heavily dependent on source and location. Ambient aerosol particles in the UK can be composed of materials including carbon, ammonium sulfate, ammonium nitrate, metals, inorganic salts such as sodium chloride, and organic materials.

For regulatory purposes particulate matter is measured in terms of mass concentration. Particulate matter varies in size. PM_{10} means the mass per cubic metre (m^3) of air of particles with a size (aerodynamic diameter) of less than 10 micrometres (μm), $PM_{2.5}$ being particles with a size generally less than 2.5 μm. Typically particles smaller than 2.5 μm diameter are referred to as fine particles and those greater than 2.5 μm diameter as coarse. Particles less than 0.1 μm (100 nanometres) are termed nanoparticles or ultrafine particles. As discussed later in the chapter, the size of the particle is important in determining the impact on health.

There are a number of sources of particulate matter in the UK as described in the following sections.

Natural sources

Natural sources of particulate matter include wind-blown dust, sea salt, particles generated from forest and bush fires, and volcanic ash. Periodically dust from the Sahara can affect air across the UK. For example, in March and April 2007 a number of monitoring stations recorded elevated concentrations of particulate matter, with many stations recording high levels of air pollution. Subsequent modelling of the prevailing air mass at the time indicated that much of the measured particulate matter originated from agricultural fires in the Ukraine and western Russia, with a contribution from sand generated by dust storms over northern Africa.

Primary or direct sources (anthropogenic)

Particulate matter can be emitted directly to air. The main sources of primary particulate matter are combustion from industries, industrial processes (for example quarrying and construction), road transport, and residential sources (for example wood and coal burning). Traffic sources can include exhaust emissions (especially from diesel vehicles), tyre and brake wear, and road surface abrasion. The introduction of cleaner engines has seen reductions in road traffic exhaust emissions and with such improvement, non-exhaust emissions (for example tyre and brake wear) are becoming more important. As a result of traffic-related particulate matter, concentrations of PM_{10} and $PM_{2.5}$ are often higher around major road networks than other urban or rural areas. Local specific sources that can be significant emitters of particles include the use of non-smokeless fuels in domestic heating and bonfires (see Case Study 4.3).

Case Study 4.3: Bonfire night 2007

In 2007, bonfire night (5 November) fell on a Monday. This led to many people holding bonfire night celebrations over the preceding weekend as well as on the traditional date itself. A high pressure weather system had settled over the north of England, resulting in low wind speeds and poor pollution dispersion. Over the weekend of 3–4 November, air monitoring stations reported elevated levels of particulate matter (measured as PM_{10}) across much of England. Northern England and the Midlands were the worst affected areas. Air pollution peaked on Sunday 4 November with 29 monitoring stations reporting values exceeding the 50 µg/m³ daily air quality objective for particulate matter. A maximum daily mean of 204 µg/m³ was recorded at the monitoring station located in Manchester Piccadilly. Wind speeds were lowest across northern England and, while short-term peaks in particulate matter were recorded in Scotland, Wales, and Northern Ireland, no exceedences of the daily standard were recorded. By 5 November, stronger winds across the north led to more favourable dispersion and lower particulate matter concentrations.

To put such an episode into context, during that weekend air pollution in parts of England were among the highest levels of particulate matter recorded in the UK for several years and fell within the 'High' to 'Very High' air quality band (see the Daily Air Quality Index section).

Secondary sources

Particulate matter can be produced by chemical reactions in the atmosphere or by condensation of gases to form solid or liquid droplets. For example, the oxidation of SO_2 and NO_x in the atmosphere produces particles composed of sulfates and nitrates. VOCs in the atmosphere can also be oxidised to form secondary particles. Measures to reduce the precursor gases such as SO_2 and NO_x can thereby reduce particulate matter to some extent. Evidence from monitoring networks in the UK indicates that secondary particles make a significant contribution to the overall background concentration of particulate matter. For example, in central and southern UK, around 60 per cent of the urban background mass of $PM_{2.5}$ is made of secondary particles (AQEG, 2012).

Regional and national/international sources

Regional or even national/international sources can be important contributors to local levels of particulate matter. Small particles can be long-lived in the atmosphere and travel many thousands of miles, and secondary particles can travel a significant distance from the original precursor source. Under certain meteorological conditions, air from continental Europe may circulate over the UK and can be a significant contributor to overall background levels of particulate matter. For example, in London a large proportion (between 40 and 50 per cent) of particulate matter originates from outside of the city but likewise particulate matter from London can affect other parts of the UK and Europe, depending on the prevailing wind direction.

Impact on health

The size of the particles is directly related to the impact on health. Particles below 10 μm in aerodynamic diameter (PM_{10}) can be inhaled into the lungs and deposited causing health problems. Coarse particles (i.e. PM_{10}) tend to be deposited in the upper airways, but fine (i.e. $PM_{2.5}$) and ultrafine particles have a higher probability of deposition deep within the lung, including on the alveoli where the uptake of oxygen occurs.

No safe threshold has been identified beneath which there are no health effects for exposure to particulate matter. Short-term (i.e. day to day) exposure to particulate matter has been linked with both cardiovascular disease and respiratory disease, and exposure to elevated levels has been associated with an increase in frequency and severity of respiratory symptoms and increased hospital admissions for treatment for cardiovascular and respiratory-related conditions. Long-term exposure to particulate matter, especially $PM_{2.5}$, has a significant impact on life expectancy, especially due to an increase in the risk of cardiovascular disease. The exact mechanism of action for this cardiovascular effect is not clear but could involve the generation of free radicals, which cause inflammation of the lungs, affecting the cardiovascular system.

Epidemiological studies have identified short- and long-term exposure to ambient levels of particulate matter to be associated with respiratory and cardiovascular illness and mortality, even at low levels. For example, studies show that long-term exposure to fine particles (monitored as $PM_{2.5}$) increases the risk of death. This finding comes from epidemiological cohort studies that compared the risk of death amongst adults aged 30 years or more living in cities or areas with high levels of $PM_{2.5}$, with the risk of death amongst those living in cities or areas with lower levels of $PM_{2.5}$. Studies (for example, Pope et al., 2004) have also identified a significantly positive association between $PM_{2.5}$ and PM_{10} and all-cause mortality and specific causes such as cardiovascular and respiratory illness.

Such epidemiological studies can allow estimation of the effect of air pollutants on mortality in the UK. The Committee on the Medical Effects of Air Pollutants (COMEAP) estimated that the burden of anthropogenic particulate matter ($PM_{2.5}$) air pollution in the UK in 2008 had an effect on mortality equivalent to 29,000 deaths at typical ages, and an associated loss of population life of 340,000 life-years (COMEAP, 2010a).

Nitrogen dioxide

Sources

The combustion of fossil fuels produces NO_x, which is the common name for a mixture of nitric oxide (NO) and nitrogen dioxide (NO_2). In most ambient situations NO is predominantly emitted and transformed in the atmosphere to NO_2 (which is more stable). The oxidation of NO to form NO_2 occurs rapidly (for example in the presence of ozone). Therefore, the highest levels of NO_2 are seen in urban areas around major road networks and it is often considered a good indicator of traffic-related pollution.

Concentrations of NO and NO_2 in ambient air have declined in the UK since the 1990s. Recently, this decline has tailed off and, in some areas, NO_2 has started to increase again. This is especially the case in urban areas and around busy roads. There are a number of reasons for this, one of which is that particulate filters on diesel vehicles are increasing the fraction of NO_2 directly emitted from the exhaust pipe. This increase in primary emissions of NO_2 has a major impact on NO_2 levels around main roads, especially in major urban areas. In many parts of the UK, legally binding EU limits for NO_2 are breached, resulting in the declaration of AQMAs.

Impact on health

At high concentrations NO_2 is an irritant that can cause inflammation of the airways. Such effects have been shown in a range of chamber studies but only at concentrations far higher than those recorded in ambient air in the UK. Some studies have suggested a link between short-term exposure to NO_2 and an increase in hospital admissions for respiratory complaints, but it is unclear whether ambient concentrations of NO_2 at current levels have a direct health effect. Some epidemiological studies have suggested that long-term exposure to ambient outdoor concentrations may have respiratory effects, especially in asthmatics and young children (WHO, 2006). However, due to the close association between NO_2 and other pollutants, such as particulate matter, it is difficult to attribute health effects solely to NO_2. As a result, it is unclear whether reported health effects from epidemiological studies are directly due to NO_2 or due to exposure to air pollutants whose concentrations correlate with those of NO_2. NO_2 contributes to the production of ozone (see Box 4.1) and secondary particulate matter, pollutants known to impact on the health of the general population.

Box 4.1 The relationship between oxides of nitrogen and ozone

Nitric oxide reacts with ozone in the atmosphere to form NO_2 by the following reaction:

$$NO + O_3 \rightarrow NO_2 + O_2$$

Therefore, in urban areas, as a result of emissions of NO_x, ozone is destroyed and NO_2 formed. However, as NO_x emissions have reduced in recent years due to emission control measures, ground level ozone concentrations are increasing.

Conversely, in the presence of sunlight, NO_2 can break down to form NO and a single oxygen atom, which can then combine with oxygen to produce ozone:

$$NO_2 + \text{sunlight} \rightarrow NO + O$$

$$O_2 + O \rightarrow O_3$$

This reaction means that in bright sunny weather, ground level ozone concentrations can increase as photolysis breaks NO_2 down to release a free oxygen atom. The three reactions outlined above form a cycle, with NO_x and O_3 existing in an equilibrium.

This equilibrium can be disturbed by the presence of other anthropogenic or naturally occurring chemicals in the atmosphere (for example CO, methane, VOCs). These substances may react in the atmosphere to form reactive chemicals that can combine with NO to form NO_2. The more NO_2 and reactive chemicals there are in the air, the more ozone will be produced in the presence of sunlight.

The chemical reactions take place over hours or days and once ozone has been generated it persists for several days. Therefore, ozone may be carried some distance away from where it was formed. Furthermore, air movement will carry NO_x emissions from their point of release (i.e. typically cities) and more ozone is then generated elsewhere, so consequently ozone concentrations rise over suburban and rural areas.

High levels of ozone occur during hot, sunny summer days with little wind and poor dispersion of air pollutants. Such conditions are well known and problematic to cities such as Athens and Los Angeles, where hills in the surrounding areas can also act to trap pollutants.

Ozone

Sources

Ground level ozone (O_3) is a gas produced by the photochemical oxidation of NO_x by sunlight (see Box 4.1), a process enhanced by the presence of VOCs. Ozone levels typically build up through the day and drop overnight, with elevated levels observed during periods of sustained high temperatures, sunshine, and light winds. Levels are typically elevated in rural and semi-rural areas and highest in the summer, often requiring the issuing of warnings and accompanying health messages to allow the population to take appropriate actions to minimise associated health effects (see Case Study 4.4).

Impact on health

Ozone is an oxidising gas that can have an irritant effect and cause inflammation in the lung. Short-term exposure to high levels results in symptoms including irritation to the eyes and nose, airway inflammation, and in severe cases, a reduction in lung function. Elevated levels have been linked with an increase in hospital admissions for respiratory disorders. Asthmatics are particularly sensitive to the effects of ozone and high levels of ozone can exacerbate asthma. However, sensitivity between individuals varies, and health studies show that ozone can have an irritant effect on both asthmatics and healthy individuals. Outdoor physical exercise may worsen the effect of ozone on lung function. Time series studies have indicated a link between ozone and mortality levels, with the number of attributable deaths brought forward estimated at 1–2 per cent on days on which the mean ozone levels reached the WHO guideline level of 100 μg/m^3 as a daily maximum 8 hour mean (WHO, 2006).

The severity of symptoms increases with ozone concentration and exposure duration. Unlike other irritant pollutants (such as SO_2), the effects of exposure build up over time; therefore, monitoring for ozone is based on an average of 8 hours as this best reflects the exposure period most likely to cause an effect. The effects of long-term exposure to ozone are not well understood. Emerging evidence suggests that long-term exposure may slow lung growth in children but further research is ongoing.

Case Study 4.4: Air quality for London 2012 Olympics

In the decade prior to the London 2012 Olympics, air quality in London improved significantly due to a number of strategic and local initiatives such as the Mayor's Air Quality Strategy for London and the government-supported Clean Air Fund. Predictions indicated that all of London would comply with most air pollution targets by 2012. However, in the run-up to the Games, air quality was identified as a concern by the International Olympic Committee (IOC), campaign groups, and the media.

The Health Protection Agency (HPA) had an important role in advising the Department of Health (DH) and the Department for Environment, Food and Rural Affairs (Defra) on the effects of air pollutants on health. The HPA worked with key stakeholders (including Defra, Greater London Authority (GLA), local authorities, air quality consultants, and academics) to provide guidance on air quality and any potential public health implications. During the Olympic and Paralympic Games, relevant air quality information was included within the public health briefings and situation reports submitted to the London Organising Committee of the Olympic and Paralympic Games (LOCOG).

Due to the warm and sunny weather, there were two episodes during the Games where air quality in the south-east of England was poor, with ozone levels recorded as 'moderate' to 'high' based on the Daily Air Quality Index. The prepared information sources and agreed procedures enabled the HPA to inform the Chief Medical Officer for the London 2012 Olympic and Paralympic Games and LOCOG in a timely and consistent manner, as well as to assist with additional questions generated by the episodes (HPA, 2013).

Fortunately, these episodes were short-lived and the organisers carefully scheduled the endurance events, such as the marathon, to avoid the mid-afternoon peaks in ozone concentration and higher temperatures.

Text extracts reproduced from Health Protection Agency, *London 2012 Olympic and Paralympic Games: Summary Report of the Health Protection Agency's Games Time Activities*, Copyright © 2013, with permission from Public Health England, available from http://www.hpa.org.uk/Topics/EmergencyResponse/2012Olympics.

Sulphur dioxide

Sources

Sulphur dioxide is produced in the environment by the combustion of sulphur-containing fossil fuels. In the UK, it is mainly emitted by industrial sources, in particular coal-fired power stations. The contribution of transport to SO_2 emissions is relatively small. Oxidation of SO_2 in the atmosphere can produce secondary particulate matter (sulfates).

Impact on health

Sulphur dioxide, a respiratory irritant, is absorbed in the upper airways and causes irritation and respiratory symptoms, including constriction of the airways of the lung and changes in pulmonary function (WHO, 2006). The effects of SO_2 can occur very rapidly, often within minutes, and monitoring is based on 15 minute averages. Susceptible individuals include those with COPD and asthmatics who are sensitive to SO_2, who can experience breathing difficulties during periods of elevated concentrations. Elevated levels have been linked with increased hospital admissions, with epidemiological studies indicating an association between 24-hour average SO_2 concentrations and deaths from cardiorespiratory causes (Maynard, 2012).

The effects of long-term exposure are not well understood. Some health studies suggest a link between long-term exposure and increased risk of mortality but, as with NO_2, it is not clear whether this is specifically due to SO_2 exposure or exposure to other pollutants.

Additional pollutants

Benzene

Benzene is a VOC. Its main sources in the environment are combustion and evaporation of petrol, industrial and domestic combustion activities, manufacturing processes (for example the use of solvents), and tobacco smoke, which can have a significant impact on indoor air quality. Benzene is a genotoxic carcinogen. Studies have shown that long-term occupational exposures to high levels of benzene can result in leukaemia. There is no safe level of exposure and consequently no safe ambient air concentration has been identified; however, levels in ambient air are much lower than those in the occupational environment. Air quality objectives for benzene are met in the UK. Levels have reduced since the 1990s, a result of the compulsory installation of catalytic convertors in motor vehicles and the reduction of the benzene content of fuels and household products such as solvents and paints.

1,3-butadiene

1,3-butadiene is a VOC, the main source of which is the combustion of petrol and diesel in motor vehicles and manufacturing activities. Like benzene, 1,3-butadiene is a genotoxic carcinogen, and there is no safe level of exposure. Occupational exposure to elevated levels over long periods has resulted in leukaemia, lymphomas, and cancer of the bone marrow and lymphoid system. In the UK, ambient levels have declined since 1990, principally as a result of the fitting of catalytic convertors to vehicle exhausts.

Carbon monoxide

Carbon monoxide is produced by the incomplete combustion of fossil fuels, for example gas and coal. The main outdoor source in the UK is road traffic emissions, in particular from petrol-driven vehicles. CO reduces the oxygen-carrying capacity of blood through the conversion of haemoglobin to carboxyhaemoglobin. Pregnant women, children, and those with cardiovascular disease are particularly vulnerable.

Exposure to low levels can result in symptoms such as headache, drowsiness, dizziness, shortness of breath, and the experience of chest pains. Exposure to elevated levels can result in neurological damage and death. Health studies suggest associations between short-term exposure to high concentrations of CO and admissions to hospital for heart attacks. There is also evidence to suggest that short- and long-term exposure can cause neurological damage.

Concentrations of CO in outdoor air are low and declining. Current monitoring suggests that they will continue to fall in the UK. Health effects are experienced at higher concentrations than those typically found in outdoor air, with indoor sources now considered a greater concern with respect to health (see Case Study 4.6).

Lead

In the UK, the common sources of lead are industrial sources such as coal combustion and iron and steel manufacturing processes. Historically the combustion of leaded fuel by motor vehicles was a major source of lead in the environment. Occupational exposure to high levels of lead can have adverse health effects, with an impact on the blood and nervous systems, kidneys, and gastrointestinal tract. No safe threshold has been identified. Pregnant women and children are particularly susceptible and chronic exposure to low levels of lead in the environment has been shown to affect children by impairing the development of their central nervous system, impacting on brain development and resulting in lower IQ, behaviour problems, and nerve damage. There has been a significant reduction in ambient air levels of lead since 1999 following the removal of lead from petrol.

Polycyclic aromatic hydrocarbons

A wide range of polycyclic aromatic hydrocarbons (PAHs) are emitted to the atmosphere from a variety of sources, typically combustion of wood and coal, industrial processes, natural fires, and traffic. Some PAHs are carcinogenic and exposure has been associated with lung cancer and tumours of the skin; however, UK ambient levels are beneath those reported to be associated with these health effects.

Indoor air quality

In the UK, air quality standards have been set to protect the population from outdoor air pollution; however, there are no similar standards for indoor air quality. The impact of indoor air quality on health is important, as in the UK people spend over 90 per cent of their time indoors (BRE, 2013).

Due to slow air exchange rates between indoor and outdoor air, there is potential for pollutants to accumulate indoors to levels that may cause adverse health effects. This problem has been exacerbated in recent years through improvements in home energy efficiency, for example by the increase in home insulation.

COMEAP made recommendations for air quality guidelines for indoor pollutants such as SO_2, NO_2, and CO (COMEAP, 2004). WHO have also produced guidelines for common indoor air pollutants (WHO Regional Office for Europe, 2010); however, these guidelines are not legally binding and there are unresolved questions about how indoor air quality should be monitored. Consequently, there is a need to improve the general public's awareness of the impact of indoor air quality on health and of how to reduce levels of indoor air pollutants, for example through ventilation of buildings and rooms, and regular maintenance of heating and cooking appliances.

The main chemical indoor air pollutants are tobacco smoke, volatile and semi-volatile organic compounds, and products of combustion. A complex mix of VOC emissions can arise from sources including building and construction materials, furnishings, paints, and glues. For example, formaldehyde, emitted by building materials such as chipboard, can cause irritation of the upper respiratory tract and eyes. Generally indoor formaldehyde levels are low; however, elevated levels associated with new building materials can have a significant impact on indoor air quality (see Case Study 4.5).

Case Study 4.5: Elevated formaldehyde levels in a school

Following the opening of a new college building, staff began to complain of symptoms such as asthma, coughing, headaches, skin irritation, sore eyes, and breathing problems. Odours were reported to be associated with these health effects. On sampling, low levels of formaldehyde were detected. While formaldehyde levels were below the WHO indoor air quality guideline, exceedences of the irritation threshold value were recorded. A site visit was undertaken and, although an odour was detectable, no source could be identified. Elevated levels could have been a result of warm rooms volatilising chemicals, highlighting the need to ventilate new build properties prior to occupancy, and the need for appropriate air exchange in educational establishments.

Build-up of CO indoors from inappropriate use of cooking or heating appliances (for example indoor use of barbeques) or poorly installed, vented, or maintained appliances can have fatal consequences. The similarity of symptoms of CO poisoning to those of flu or food poisoning often delays proper diagnosis. In England and Wales, approximately 40 deaths a year result from acute exposure to CO. The burden of disease associated with chronic exposure to low levels of carbon monoxide is currently unknown (Cross Government Group on Gas Safety and CO awareness, 2012). CO can also be produced by the incomplete combustion of coal, coke, oil, wood, and charcoal (see Case Study 4.6).

Case Study 4.6: Residential CO poisoning associated with a restaurant

Over a period of 3 months, residents in a flat were repeatedly alerted to elevated CO levels by their CO detector. The installation of monitoring equipment within the restaurant below and the flat confirmed a correlation between CO concentrations, with CO levels rising within the restaurant in the late evening, followed by a rise in concentrations in the flat above. The charcoal-fired tandoor oven in the restaurant was identified as the source. Smouldering charcoal was left burning overnight with the air extraction system turned off. The inadequate ventilation led to a build-up of CO within the restaurant and the neighbouring flat above.

This, and a number of similar recent cases, illustrates the need to consider neighbouring sources during a CO investigation, as CO can infiltrate through walls and floors, and consequently neighbours can be at risk from appliances in adjacent properties. This can complicate identification of a source, leading to delays in the recognition of the problem, reporting, and intervention by the appropriate authorities.

Health burden resulting from ambient air pollution

The symptoms and magnitude of health effects that may be observed following exposure to air pollutants are often represented as a pyramid (Figure 4.1). Less frequent, more severe health outcomes, such as death from respiratory disease, are at the top of the pyramid, with conditions that will lead to reduced quality of life further down, through to frequent, less severe outcomes such as minor irritation at the bottom. An individual's sensitivity to a pollutant could lead to a more severe response following exposure and specific outcomes (for example hospital admission) could occur at lower pollutant concentrations.

Nobody knows how many deaths are in part, or wholly, caused by environmental pollutants. Individual pollutants could be associated with a wide range of health effects, and few diseases are directly attributable to a single pollutant. Some pollutants may only affect individuals after prolonged or repeated exposure. Pollutants may also interact with each other, or with other environmental factors such as temperature or airborne allergens, to act synergistically and produce a health effect. All these factors can create difficulties in considering and determining associations between environmental pollution and health.

As stated earlier, the burden (effect) of long-term exposure to anthropogenic $PM_{2.5}$ air pollution in the UK in 2008 was estimated to be equivalent to nearly 29,000 deaths at typical ages (COMEAP, 2010a). This represents a loss of life expectancy from birth of approximately 6 months in England. There are uncertainties associated with this estimate; the burden could be lower but it could equally be higher. Air pollution is unlikely to be the sole cause of death and it may be that air pollution was a contributory factor in a larger number of deaths, just as other risk factors (for example diets high in fat or sugar and lack of exercise) may contribute.

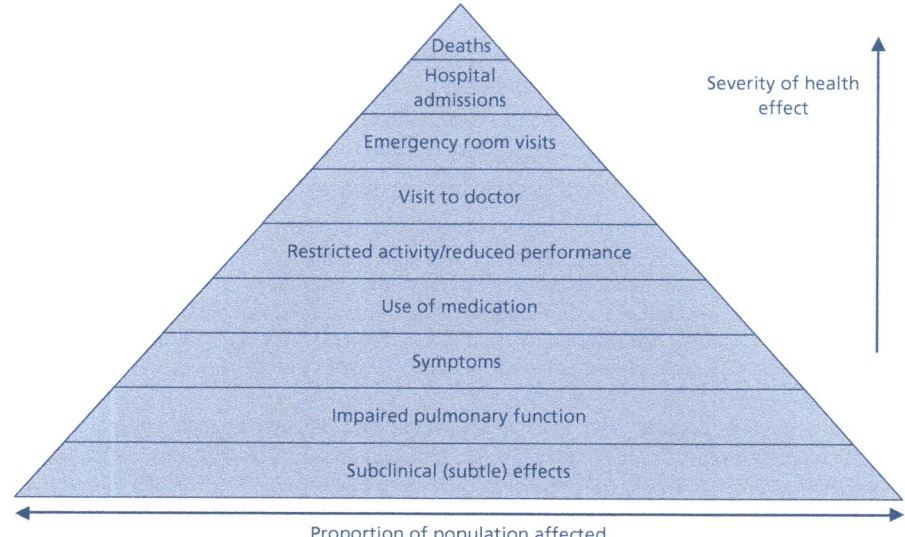

Fig. 4.1 Air pollution health effects pyramid.

Reproduced from World Health Organization Regional Office for Europe, *Quantification of the Health Effects of Exposure to Air Pollution: Report of a WHO Working Group, Bilthoven, Netherlands, 20–22 November 2000*, Copyright © 2001, with permission from the World Health Organization, available from http://www.euro.who.int/en/what-we-do/health-topics/environment-and-health/air-quality/publications/pre2009/quantification-of-health-effects-of-exposure-to-air-pollution. Source: Data from American Thoracic Society (ATS), What constitutes an adverse health effect of air pollution? *American Journal of Respiratory and Critical Care Medicine*, Volume 161, Issue 2, pp. 665–673, Copyright © 2000 The American Thoracic Society.

The quantification of health impacts is based on the mortality burden associated with exposure to long-term $PM_{2.5}$; however, air pollution also affects morbidity and air pollution-related illnesses are likely to have an additional health burden. Similarly, there will be a mortality burden from short-term exposure to other pollutants (for example ozone), although these are likely to be less significant.

It has been estimated that removing all anthropogenic fine particulate air pollution would have a bigger impact on life expectancy in England and Wales than eliminating passive smoking or road traffic accidents (Miller and Hurley, 2006). To put this into perspective, the economic cost from the health impacts of air pollution in the UK is estimated at £8.5–20.2 billion every year (Defra, 2007), compared to the economic cost of obesity of £5 billion per year (DH, 2011). However, everyone in the population is exposed to air pollution; it is not a lifestyle choice.

Air pollution as a public health indicator

There are many factors that influence public health over the course of a lifetime. The integration of public health into local government (in 2013) will allow these factors to be considered in a holistic manner, with services planned and delivered in the context of the broader social determinants of health, including poverty, education, housing, employment, crime, and pollution. In England, a Public Health Outcomes Framework sets out a vision for public health, defining 68 indicators to improve understanding of the success of public health interventions. One of these indicators relates to air quality and represents an estimate of the effect of long-term exposure to current levels of anthropogenic particulate air pollution on adult mortality. The estimate is expressed as a fraction (percentage) of total (all-cause) adult mortality attributable to long-term exposure to current levels of anthropogenic particulate air pollution in the different local authority areas (i.e. the estimate is a health burden equivalent to a specified proportion of all deaths occurring annually in the region under consideration). This indicator is calculated from population-weighted modelled concentrations of fine particulate matter ($PM_{2.5}$) in air at background (for example not roadside) locations in 2010 in each of the upper tier local authority areas in England. A concentration-response coefficient linking ambient $PM_{2.5}$ concentrations with an increased mortality risk in adults aged over 30 is used to estimate mortality.

This indicator is one of three measures recommended by COMEAP to estimate mortality from $PM_{2.5}$ at a local level. The other two metrics are attributable death, and associated years of life lost by the local population.

Such indicators can provide information about the impact locally of air pollution on public health, which can be compared with other factors detrimental to public health. This should allow appropriate priority to be given to actions to reduce the exposure of the local population to air pollution. Decreasing air pollution can contribute to increasing healthy life expectancy and reducing early death from cardiovascular and respiratory diseases. In addition, there are a number of other indicators that could benefit from measures taken to improve air quality. For example, policies and activities that increase the use of public transport and encourage people to walk or cycle on journeys for which they would previously have used the car would also contribute towards a number of NHS and public health outcomes (such as reduction of mortality from respiratory disease, cardiovascular disease, and so on), as well as towards a reduction in greenhouse gas emissions.

Daily Air Quality Index

The Daily Air Quality Index (DAQI) is a banding system recommended by COMEAP and used in the UK to communicate information about air pollution via the Defra UK Air Information Resource web pages. The index provides daily real-time and predicted forecasts on short-term levels of air pollution concentrations, in terms of index bands (numbered 1–10). These bands provide an indication of potential health effects associated with these levels for susceptible groups (i.e. those with lung problems, asthma, and adults with health conditions) and the general public, similar to the pollen or sun index (see Table 4.2). Advanced warning of poor air quality and accompanying health messages for at-risk individuals and the general public allows individuals to easily determine whether they are at risk and whether they need to undertake actions, such as avoiding strenuous activity or more frequent use of treatment (for example inhalers) to minimise associated health effects.

Table 4.2 DAQI bandings and associated actions that may be needed at each level

Air quality index category	Recommended action
Low (1–3)	At-risk individuals and general population are unlikely to suffer adverse health effects associated with air pollution and should enjoy usual outdoor activities.
Moderate (4–6)	Potential for susceptible individuals, for example those with lung or heart conditions, to experience symptoms. Those who experience symptoms should consider reducing strenuous physical activity. The healthy general population should enjoy outdoor activities as usual.
High (7–9)	Associated with significant health effects in susceptible individuals. Susceptible individuals should consider reducing strenuous activity, and the general population should consider reducing activities if symptoms are experienced.
Very High (10)	Susceptible individuals and the general population may experience adverse health effects. Susceptible individuals should avoid strenuous activities at this level, and the general population should consider reducing physical exertion, especially in the presence of symptoms such as a cough or sore throat.

Reproduced from Department for Environment, Food and Rural Affairs (Defra), *The Air Quality Index* © Crown Copyright 2013, licence under the under the Open Government Licence v1.0, available from: http://uk-air.defra.gov.uk/air-pollution/daqi.

The index is based on the health effects of short-term exposure to the following pollutants, with the pollution index defined by the highest concentration of pollutant over the next 24 hours:

- nitrogen dioxide (NO_2)
- sulphur dioxide (SO_2)
- ozone (O_3)
- fine particulate matter ($PM_{2.5}$)
- coarse particulate matter (PM_{10})

The index is divided into four air quality categories indicating the level of air pollution, which are then divided in a ten-point scale to provide greater detail of air pollution levels.

Air pollution mitigation measures

The resultant air quality at any location and time will depend on a number of factors, including:

- the quantity and type of pollutants emitted from natural and anthropogenic sources
- topography (terrain), such as urban streets, rural areas, mountains, and valleys
- weather, such as wind, temperature, air turbulence, air pressure, rainfall, and cloud cover
- the physical and chemical properties of pollutants and atmospheric processes such as dry and wet deposition and photochemical reactions.

When implementing mitigation measures for air pollution, it is important to recognise and consider climate change issues. Air pollution and greenhouse gas emissions arise from similar sources and they can benefit from emission reduction strategies, resulting in greater combined benefits than tackling the issues separately. However, trade-offs may be necessary where actions on one issue have a negative impact on the other.

Emission reduction schemes: low emission zones

In most urban cities in the UK, road transport is the dominant source of air pollution and the proximity of people and residential properties to busy urban roads has led to the declaration of many AQMAs. The spatial design and use of urban areas together with transportation need to be considered when seeking improvements in air quality. Transport associated with construction, occupation, and use of new developments can lead to transport emissions (and/or an increase in human exposure to transport-related air pollutants). In contrast, well designed developments may actively help to enhance air quality, manage exposure, and reduce overall emissions (Defra, 2010).

Therefore, it is important to recognise the interactions and role that land use and transport planning can have in air quality at the local, regional, and national level. Low emission strategies, which complement other development and transport policies and strategies, can provide a package of measures to help mitigate the transport impacts of the urban environment and its development. For example, measures could include encouraging a reduction in vehicle use, a modal shift towards sustainable transport, or aiding the accelerated uptake of cleaner fuels (for example through provision of low emission infrastructure and incentives for take-up). Many local authorities (singularly and together) have prepared low emissions strategies.

Low emission zones (LEZs) are an example of a low emission strategy used in cities to tackle air pollutants. They are primarily focussed on reducing fine particulate matter and NO_2. LEZs are defined as geographical areas where vehicles are restricted from entering, or discouraged through the implementation of a charge, if their emissions are over a set level. The restriction of older, more polluting vehicles in a LEZ can encourage the turnover of the fleet (or, if feasible, the fitting of abatement equipment). Traffic volumes may not necessarily change; however, as vehicles travelling within the designated area have lower emissions, air quality improvements should be seen. The LEZ can apply to any clearly identifiable and reasonable categorisation, for example engine size, Euro emissions category, carbon dioxide emissions, vehicle age, class, or weight, fuel type, or a combination of these (Kilbane-Dawe, 2012). An example of a LEZ established for London is given in Case Study 4.7.

In 2008, PM_{10} from vehicles made up around 79 per cent of the total emissions in central London; this is predicted to be 75 per cent by 2015. Road transport also contributes a significant proportion of NO_x emissions (approximately 60 per cent), although throughout London as a whole the contribution is lower due to the greater presence of other sources (for example industry, rail, and airports). The Mayor's Air Quality Strategy (MAQS) (GLA, 2010) sets out a number of measures to tackle air pollution, in particular from traffic sources, including the introduction of hybrid diesel-electric buses, the promotion of a modal shift towards cleaner forms of transport (for example encouraging the uptake of electric and other low emission vehicles), the operation of a low emission zone, and the provision of an infrastructure to encourage walking and cycling.

Case Study 4.7: London Low Emission Zone

Commencing in 2008, in order to drive within the zone without paying a daily charge, heavy goods vehicles, lorries, buses, and coaches were required to meet Euro III emissions standards for particulate matter and then, by 2012, the more stringent Euro IV standards. The LEZ operates 24 hours a day, 356 days per year and its geographical extent is shown in Figure 4.2.

Further restrictions to vehicle emissions within the LEZ are planned to help to reduce NO_x concentrations; by the end of 2015 the Transport for London bus fleet operating within the zone will be Euro IV or more stringent. The London LEZ covers an area in which more than 8 million people live and work, and includes areas with the highest exceedences of air pollution in Greater London (Kelly et al., 2011). At 2644 m² and encompassing most of Greater London, this LEZ is one of the largest in the world. In 2013, the Mayor of London announced plans to develop the LEZ further to create an Ultra-Low Emission Zone in central London by 2020.

Are LEZs effective at improving air quality and do they result in a positive impact on public health outcomes? A review of the London LEZ (Kelly et al., 2011) predicted modest

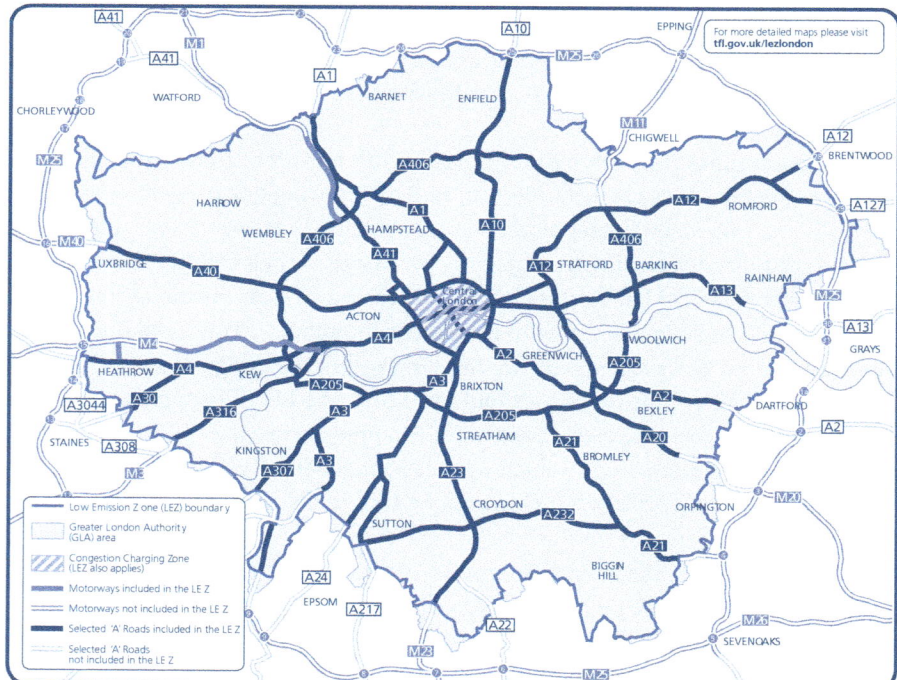

Fig. 4.2 The geographical extent of the London Low Emission Zone (TfL).

Reproduced with permission from Transport for London (TfL), Copyright © Transport for London 2013.

reductions (of around 3–7 per cent) in total emissions for PM_{10}, NO_x, and NO_2 between 2008 and 2012. Similar emission reductions were predicted or determined for environmental zones (or low emission zones) in other cities and countries (for example Rome, Germany, and The Netherlands) (Boogaard, 2012; Ceseroni et al., 2012; Malina and Fischer, 2012). The London LEZ review also considered health records, estimating that a 5 to10 per cent reduction in respiratory illness consultations or prescriptions for asthma would occur for patients most exposed to the intervention compared with patients presumed not to be exposed to it (Kelly et al., 2011).

Removal of pollutants from ambient air

Recently, consideration has been given to measures that can be used to remove pollutants from ambient air. For example, particulate matter can be trapped through the use of a chemical-based dust suppressant such as calcium magnesium acetate (CMA), which, when applied to roadways or building facades, can lead to reductions in dust and particulate re-suspension.

Green space and natural features in the urban environment, including street trees, gardens, green roofs, green or living walls, and green screens, all make up the green infrastructure of our urban areas. Vegetation and trees in urban green space can influence air quality in a number of ways; for example, through direct absorption of gaseous pollutants and interception of particles onto leaf surfaces, by lowering air temperatures through transpiration, which can reduce the formation of ozone, and through the direct production of oxygen during photosynthesis (Forest Research, 2010). The ability of plants to capture air pollutants depends on the size, shape, and surface texture of leaves. For example, particulates are effectively trapped by leaves that are hairy, rough, and/or ridged. Vegetation with small leaves provides a greater density of foliage, branches, and leaf area on which to absorb particles. Plants that attract aphids could also be beneficial as the sticky secretion of aphids deposited on leaves will aid the retention of particles (TfL, 2012).

It is estimated that vegetation in urban areas currently removes 1 to 5 per cent of particulate matter and gaseous pollutants (Nowak et al., 2006; Pugh et al., 2012). However, it is estimated that effective land use planning and further 'greening' of urban areas could increase this significantly. Whilst green infrastructure can be used as a supplementary measure to reduce air pollution, it has also been demonstrated to provide wider environmental and health benefits, including increasing biodiversity, aiding climate change adaption and mitigation, and improving health and wellbeing (encouraging physical activity and reducing stress and health inequalities). Furthermore, children living near street trees are found to have a lower prevalence of childhood asthma (Forest Research, 2010; Lovasi et al., 2008).

Individual intervention measures

Air quality in the UK has significantly improved over the past 50 years and pollutant concentrations are normally described as 'low' or at the lower end of the 'moderate' band within the DAQI. For the majority of the time, even sensitive individuals will not notice an effect of air pollution on their health.

Air quality intervention services (such as airTEXT, airAware, airAlert, and 'Know and Respond') provide free information about air pollution and related health advice to anyone wishing to know about the quality of the air they breathe. These services are of particular benefit to people with medical conditions that may be affected or exacerbated by air pollution, such as asthma, emphysema, chronic bronchitis, heart disease, or angina (see Case Study 4.8). The services allow users to take steps to modify their behaviour and take action to help reduce the likelihood of any impacts. For example, vulnerable recipients are able to make a decision not to exercise outside during periods of high pollution, or to make sure they carry extra medication with them. This empowers and enables individuals to manage their health conditions more effectively.

Case Study 4.8: Alerting and awareness raising

Air quality intervention and early warning systems are designed to alert users, via a range of media (for example voice message, text message, email, mobile phone app), when air pollution levels are predicted to be elevated. The London Borough of Croydon established the airTEXT service in 2005, which now operates London-wide. In 2011–2012, the service was further developed to provide daily information on air quality, predicted pollen levels, UV radiation levels, and temperature, with a daily health bulletin produced for health, leisure, and tourism venues across London for use during the 2012 Olympic and Paralympic Games.

There is also a need to raise public awareness of air quality issues and for ongoing local and regional efforts to highlight actions individuals can undertake to improve air quality or reduce their exposure to air pollution. There are a number of awareness-raising groups and campaigns in England. For example, Care4Air is a partnership between four local authorities in South Yorkshire, funded by the South Yorkshire Local Transport Plan. It aims to raise awareness of air quality issues and encourage behaviour that helps to reduce air pollution. As a portal it provides information on regional initiatives to individuals, local businesses, schools, and organisations, with information and tools to enable everyone to 'do their bit'.

Research on the airTEXT and airAlert intervention services have shown that subscribers have a better understanding of the relationship between environmental triggers and their symptoms and are therefore more prepared and better able to plan their activities (Smallbone, 2009), thereby potentially reducing the number of acute health effects and decreasing the financial burden on the NHS.

Alternatives to the use of vehicles

National and local transportation and planning policies that promote a modal shift in travel towards walking and cycling can further contribute to combating air pollution. Like other forms of transport, there are risks associated with walking and cycling such as the risk of injury from falls or collisions and exposure to air pollution. However, the benefits to health of increased physical activity outweigh these dis-benefits. Other potential co-benefits of a modal shift towards physically active travel include reductions in noise, congestion, and emissions of carbon dioxide (a greenhouse gas).

Every year in the UK, the average person makes about 46 car journeys of less than a mile, either as a driver or passenger. Some of these journeys by car are a necessity; however, studies show that a proportion of these are made because time is short, the journey is considered 'a long way', or it is more convenient. It is estimated that, with a little planning, about one car journey a month could probably be walked or cycled instead. By choosing walking or cycling as an alternative, overall levels of physical activity are likely to be increased, which can contribute towards a number of health benefits (NICE, 2012):

- reducing the risk of coronary heart disease, stroke, cancer, obesity, and type 2 diabetes
- keeping the musculoskeletal system healthy
- promoting mental wellbeing.

Although it may be theoretically possible for journeys, particularly local trips, to be made using alternative modes of travel, there are barriers that prevent the switch being made. Infrastructure issues (for example motor traffic volume and speed, lack of convenient road crossings, poorly maintained footpaths or cycleways, and so on) can discourage people from walking and cycling. More thought and preparation may be needed prior to starting a journey and journey times may be longer. Through implementation of local initiatives, individuals and communities can be encouraged to choose alternative modes of travel. A few examples are provided below:

- Town or city-wide activity programmes to promote cycling for both transport and recreational purposes. These include cycle hire schemes, car-free days, provision of maps, and route signing.
- Schools and workplaces could encourage their communities and staff to be more physically active, for example, through the organization of cycle to work/school days or weeks.
- Integration of walking routes with public transport links to support longer journeys. Tools such as the 'walkit' website, an interactive urban journey planner, can demonstrate how walking can replace all or part of any given journey, including those to work or school, as well as identifying routes away from busy roads to help reduce personal exposure to air pollution.

Incidents and emerging air quality issues

Fires and air pollution

Smoke comprises a complex mixture of particles and gases. Large fires can cause air pollution episodes through the generation of a smoke plume consisting of gaseous pollutants and solid and liquid particulate matter. Given the complex and varied nature of materials that may be involved in a fire, potentially a wide range of pollutants can be released in a smoke plume. It is extremely difficult to state with any certainty exactly what a smoke plume may contain. Different materials release different pollutants upon combustion and typically there is considerable uncertainty about the exact composition of the materials involved in the fire. As well as variations in emissions due to the nature of the material involved, the composition of the smoke will vary depending on the nature of the fire, the temperature of combustion, and the availability of oxygen for the combustion process. Efficient, well oxygenated fires, for example, produce smoke containing less complex organic components than low temperature, smouldering fires, whilst incomplete combustion of organic material generates carbonaceous particles. These may contain a range of metals, depending on the fuel, and organic compounds, including polycyclic aromatic hydrocarbon (PAH) compounds. Additionally, chemical conversions occur both during combustion and as products of combustion enter the wider environment during and after the fire; for example, chemicals may react on mixing with water during firefighting activities or through reactions in the combustion zone.

There is a small but growing evidence base on emissions from fires. For example, fires involving large quantities of rubber, such as tyre fires, can generate significant yields of sulphur dioxide due to the high sulphur content resulting from the vulcanisation process, as well as particles, CO, organic and inorganic irritants, PAHs, and organic compounds such as benzene, styrene, phenols, and butadiene (Shakya et al., 2008).

In toxicological terms smoke may be considered as comprising a mixture of particulate matter, largely carbon but including other substances and gases (for example CO and hydrogen cyanide). Smoke is acutely irritating to the eyes, nose, and upper airways. This effect is caused by particles and also by volatile compounds such as acrolein and SO_2. High concentrations of certain constituents, for example, CO, hydrogen cyanide, and phosgene, can cause acute poisoning leading to collapse and death. Typically these effects result from the high concentrations that occur in a building that is on fire, especially if the fire is smouldering.

Smoke from fires can have a measurable health effect. For example, forest and bush-fires have caused sustained air quality problems in many countries and have been associated with admissions to hospital for respiratory problems (Chen et al., 2006; Tham et al., 2009). In the UK, exposure to prolonged periods of poor air quality from fires is rare but they do occasionally occur, and in recent years such fires have typically involved waste processing facilities (see Case Study 4.9).

Case Study 4.9: Waste tyre fire that impacted on local air quality

In 2009, a tyre fire resulted in daily exceedances of the UK Air Quality Objective for particulate matter over a 10 day period. The fire involved scrap tyres and produced a dense black plume of smoke that slowly dispersed over the local town (population of 5000). Air monitoring was undertaken at a number of locations downwind of the fire. Shelter advice to the public was tailored based on forecasted modelling predictions of the plume direction, observations at the scene with regard to the dispersion of smoke, and locations of susceptible groups of people within the town (for example schoolchildren). This information was also used to support decisions regarding firefighting activities at the scene, to minimise the production of smoke and the impact on the local community.

The most common approach to reducing exposure to raised concentrations of airborne pollutants from events such as fires is to shelter. Individuals are advised to remain indoors with their windows and doors closed until outdoor concentrations fall. This is prudent short-term advice. Pollutants generated outdoors will, of course, infiltrate into buildings over time but peak concentrations indoors are likely to be significantly lower than outdoors. Most studies suggest an indoor and outdoor ratio of pollutant concentrations (I/O) of between 0.6 and 0.7. This is valuable especially as regards avoiding the effects of irritant compounds where health effects are associated with acute exposure. Time-series studies tend to consider only 24-hour average concentrations and provide no information on the possible importance of peak concentrations within the 24-hour period. This caveat applies probably even more strongly to the data produced by cohort studies; areas with high long-term average concentrations are likely to experience high short-term average concentrations but the effects of time cannot be deduced from the study results. Sheltering can only be a short-term measure; people cannot be expected to stay indoors for weeks or months.

Evacuation of people from danger areas carries a significant risk. This is imposed by the stress of evacuation and temporary, often makeshift accommodation, and by the physical risks associated with the process. Evacuation is considered a last resort and will, almost always, be advised rather than imposed. Incidents in which an area is evacuated are rare and are more likely to be a result of an obvious and severe risk, for example, explosive risk resulting from the presence of gas cylinders or a leaking gas main, rather than the risks imposed by the impact of smoke blowing across a residential area. Voluntary evacuation is a more common response and consequently those at greatest risk should be identified and tailored advice provided. In principle, those with known cardio-respiratory disease and those in frail health, including a proportion of the elderly, are at greatest risk. Balancing the risks associated with exposure to smoke and those associated with evacuation is difficult and cannot be done in a satisfactorily quantitative way.

Ultrafine particulate matter

Ultrafine particulate matter is particulate matter with a diameter of less than 100 nm. Sources include combustion processes, in particular diesel vehicle emissions, and due to the recent emergence of nanotechnology as a novel area of research, ultrafine particles, otherwise known as nanoparticles, are increasingly used in a wide variety of technologies, including medicine and electronics (Kumar et al., 2010). Consequently the population is exposed to a wide variety of ultrafine particles on a daily basis and this extensive use has led to heightened concerns due to the limited knowledge of their impact on health. Discussions of the impact that PM_{10} and $PM_{2.5}$ have on health have highlighted the role these particles play. Due to their small size they are able to migrate from the site of deposition into the blood. As with PM_{10}, there is concern due to the potential for oxidative stress and inflammatory response resulting from exposure; however, research is ongoing to characterise the impact of exposure to these particles on health.

Climate change and air pollution

Climate change can have implications for regional air quality as rising temperatures may affect ozone levels and consequently human health. Natural emissions of ozone precursors, such as isoprene from vegetation, generally increase as the climate warms. Changes in soil moisture associated with climate change will also influence dry deposition of ozone, leading to higher concentrations as soils become drier in summer.

A recent modelling study has indicated that a uniform 5°C increase in temperature over the UK would lead to an increase in annual mean ozone of nearly 3 µg/m^3 (6 µg/m^3 in the summer) in south-east England. However, it should be noted that changes in ozone concentrations due to climate change are likely to be smaller than potential changes due to future changes in ozone precursor emissions (for example oxides of nitrogen and volatile organic compounds) in the UK and abroad, or due to inter-annual variability in weather conditions (Vardoulakis and Heaviside, 2012).

Climate change may also affect ambient concentrations of other air pollutants through changes in atmospheric transport and mixing processes. Measures to mitigate and adapt to climate change, for example, reduced use of private cars, reduced use of fossil fuels for energy generation, and improved thermal insulation of houses, could provide local air quality and public health co-benefits, as well as reducing greenhouse gas emissions.

Summary

In the UK, ambient air pollution has decreased significantly in recent decades; however, it is still a significant public health issue and high levels of certain pollutants are known to be responsible for adverse health effects. For example, short-term exposures can result in the exacerbation of pre-existing conditions such as cardiovascular and respiratory diseases, leading to the need for treatment and increased hospital admissions. Epidemiological studies have been instrumental in providing evidence linking health effects and exposure to ambient levels of air pollution; however, further work is required in order to fully understand and quantify the health burden associated with these pollutants.

Legislation, technological advances (for example redesigning vehicle engines and improving fuels), and novel measures such as the implementation of low emission zones have all led to significant improvements in air quality. Improvements such as these will have a direct benefit to public health by, for example, increasing healthy life expectancy.

Acknowledgement

We gratefully acknowledge the contribution of Sotiris Vardoulakis in reviewing the chapter and the case studies provided by Catherine Keshishian and Charlotte Landeg-Cox.

References

Air Quality Expert Group (AQEG) (2012). *Fine Particulate Matter (PM2.5) in the United Kingdom*. Available at: https://www.gov.uk/government/uploads/system/uploads/attachment_data/file/69635/pb13837-aqeg-fine-particle-matter-20121220.pdf [Accessed 10 April 2013].

Boogaard, H. (2012). *Effects of Traffic Policies on Air Pollution and Health—An intervention study*. Thesis Utrecht University, ISBN: 978-90-393-5830-6. Available at: http://igitur-archive.library.uu.nl/dissertations/2012-0913-200556/Manuscript-definitief.pdf [Accessed 10 April 2013].

Buildings Research Establishment (BRE) (2013). Indoor Air Quality [website]. Available at: http://www.bre.co.uk/page.jsp?id=720 [Accessed 24 May 2013].

Ceseroni, G., Boogaard, H., Jonkers, S., Porta, D., Badaloni, C., Cattani, G., et al. (2012). Health benefits of traffic-related air pollution reduction in different socioeconomic groups: the effect of low-emission zoning in Rome. *Occupational and Environmental Medicine*, **69**, 133–139.

Chen, L., Verrall, K., and Tong, S. (2006). Air particulate pollution due to bushfires and respiratory hospital admissions in Brisbane, Australia. *International Journal of Environmental Health Research*, **16:**3, 181–191.

Committee on the Medical Effects of Air Pollutants (COMEAP) (2004). *Guidance on the Effects on Health of Indoor Air Pollutants*. Available at: http://www.comeap.org.uk/documents/reports/39-page-linking/page-linking/67-indoor-air-pollutants [Accessed 11 April 2013].

Committee on the Medical Effects of Air Pollutants (COMEAP) (2010a). *The Mortality Effects of Long-Term Exposure to Particulate Air Pollution in the United Kingdom*. Available at: http://www.comeap.org.uk/documents/reports [Accessed 10 April 2013].

Committee on the Medical Effects of Air Pollution (COMEAP) (2010b). *COMEAP Statement: Does Outdoor Air Pollution Cause Asthma?* Available at: http://www.comeap.org.uk/documents/statements/39-page/linking/53-does-outdoor-air-pollution-cause-asthma [Accessed 23 May 2013].

Cross Government Group on Gas Safety and Carbon monoxide (CO) awareness (2012). *Annual Report 2011/2012*. Available at: http://www.hse.gov.uk/gas/domestic/cross-government-group-1112.pdf [Accessed 24 May 2013].

Department for Environment, Food and Rural Affairs (Defra) (2007). *The Air Quality Strategy for England, Scotland, Wales and Northern Ireland (Volume 1)*. HMSO, London.

Department for Environment, Food and Rural Affairs (Defra) (2009). *Local Air Quality Management Technical Guidance LAQM.TG(09)*. Available at: https://www.gov.uk/government/uploads/system/uploads/attachment_data/file/69334/pb13081-tech-guidance-laqm-tg-09-090218.pdf [Accessed 10 April 2013].

Department for Environment, Food and Rural Affairs (Defra) (2010). *Low Emissions Strategies: Using the planning system to reduce transport emissions*. Good Practice Guidance, January 2010. Available at: http://www.lowemissionstrategies.org/downloads/LES_Good_Practice_Guide_2010.pdf [Accessed 20 May 2013].

Department for Environment, Food and Rural Affairs (Defra) (2013) The Air Quality Index [website]. Available at: http://uk-air.defra.gov.uk/air-pollution/daqi [Accessed 12 April 2013].

Department of Health (DH) (2011). *Healthy Lives, Healthy People: A call to action on obesity in England*. Available at: https://www.gov.uk/government/publications/healthy-lives-healthy-people-a-call-to-action-on-obesity-in-england [Accessed 28 May 2013].

Department of Health (2012). *An Outcomes Strategy for COPD and Asthma: NHS Companion Document*. Available at: https://www.gov.uk/government/publications/an-outcomes-strategy-for-copd-and-asthma-nhs-companion-document [Accessed 10 April 2013].

Forest Research (2010). *Benefits of Green Infrastructure. Report by Forest Research*. Forest Research, Farnham. Available at: http://www.forestry.gov.uk/pdf/urgp_benefits_of_green_infrastructure.pdf/$file/urgp_benefits_of_green_infrastructure.pdf [Accessed 10 April 2013].

Greater London Authority (GLA) (2010). *Clearing the Air. The Mayor's Air Quality Strategy*. December 2010. Available at: http://www.london.gov.uk/priorities/environment/publications/mayors-air-quality-strategy [Accessed 10 April 2013].

Health Protection Agency (HPA) (2013). *London 2012 Olympic and Paralympic Games: Summary Report of the Health Protection Agency's Games Time Activities*. Available at: http://www.hpa.org.uk/Topics/EmergencyResponse/2012Olympics/ [Accessed 5 April 2013].

Kelly, F., Armstrong, B., Atkinson, R., Anderson, H. R., Barratt, B., Beevers, S., et al. (2011). *The London Low Emission Zone Baseline Study; with critique from the HEI Health Review Committee,*

Research Report 163. Health Effects Institute (HEI), Boston, Massachusetts. Available at: http://pubs.healtheffects.org/view.php?id=366 [Accessed 10 April 2013].

Kilbane-Dawe, I. (2012). *14 Cost Effective Actions to Cut Central London Air Pollution*. Release 2 (31.7.2012). Par Hill Research Ltd, London.

Kumar, P., Robins, A., Vardoulakis, S., and Britter, R. (2010). A review of the characteristics of nanoparticles in the urban atmosphere and the prospects for developing regulatory controls. *Atmospheric Environment*, **44**, 5035–5052.

Lovasi, G. S., Quinn, J. W., Neckerman, K. M., Perzanowski, M. S., and Rundle, A. (2008). Children living in areas with more street trees have lower prevalence of asthma. *Journal of Epidemiology and Community Health*, **62**, 647–649.

Malina, C. and Fischer, F. (2012). *The Impact of Low Emission Zones on PM_{10} Levels in Urban Areas in Germany*. CAWM Discussion Paper No. 58, University of Muenster, 20 August 2012. Available at: http://www.wiwi.uni-muenster.de/cawm/forschen/Download/The-impact-of-low-emission-zones-on-PM10-levels-in-urban-areas-in-Germany.pdf [Accessed 10 April 2013].

Maynard, R. (2012). Air pollution in the United Kingdom. In: Baker, D., Karalliedde, L., Murray, V., Maynard, R., and Parkinson, N. (Eds) 2nd ed. *Essentials of Toxicology for Health Protection: A Handbook for field professionals*, pp 111–124. Oxford University Press, Oxford.

Miller, B. G. and Hurley, J. F. (2006). *Comparing Estimated Risks for Air Pollution with Risks for Other Health Effects*. Institute of Occupational Medicine (IOM). Available at: http://www.iom-world.org/pubs/IOM_TM0601.pdf [Accessed 28 May 2013].

National Institute for Clinical Excellence (NICE) (2012). *Walking and Cycling: Local measures to promote walking and cycling as forms of travel or recreation*. Available at: http://publications.nice.org.uk/walking-and-cycling-local-measures-to-promote-walking-and-cycling-as-forms-of-travel-or-recreation-ph41 [Accessed 20 May 2013].

Nowak, D. J., Crane, D. E., and Stevens, J. C. (2006). Air pollution removal by urban trees and shrubs in the United States. *Urban Forestry and Urban Greening*, **4**, 115–123.

Pope, C. A. III., Burnett, R. T., Thurston, G. D., Thun, M. J., Calle, E. E., Krewski, D. et al. (2004). Cardiovascular mortality and long term exposure to particulate air pollution. *Circulation*, **109**, 71–77.

Pugh, T. A. M, MacKenzie, A. R., Whyatt, J. D., and Hewitt, C. N. (2012). Effectiveness of green infrastructure for improvement of air quality in urban street canyons. *Environmental Science and Technology*, **46**, 7692–7699.

Shakya, P. R., Shrestha, P., Tamrakar, C. S., and Bhattarai, P. K. (2008). Studies on potential emission of hazardous gases due to uncontrolled open-air burning of waste vehicle tyres and their possible impacts on the environment. *Atmospheric Environment*, **42**, 6555–6565.

Smallbone, K. (2009). Direct delivery of predicted air pollution information to people with respiratory illness: an evaluation. In: Health Protection Agency (HPA) *Chemical Hazards and Poisons Report September 2009*, Issue 15, pp 32–34. Available at: http://www.hpa.org.uk/Publications/ChemicalsPoisons/ChemicalHazardsAndPoisonsReports/ [Accessed 10 April 2013].

Tham, R., Erbas, B., Akram, M., Dennekamp, M., and Abramson, M. J. (2009). The impact of smoke on respiratory hospital outcomes during the 2002–2003 bushfire season, Victoria, Australia. *Respirology*, **14**, 69–75.

Transport for London (TfL) (2012). *Delivering Vertical Greening. Project Review. October 2012*. Available at: http://www.london.gov.uk/sites/default/files/2012-10-15%20Delivering%20Vertical%20Greening.pdf [Accessed 10 April 2013].

Transport for London (TfL) (2013) Emissions standards have changed. Have you taken action? [website]. Available at: http://www.tfl.gov.uk/assets/downloads/roadusers/lez/lez-leaflet-jan-2012.pdf [Accessed 10 April 2013].

Vardoulakis, S. and Heaviside, C. (Eds) (2012). *Health Effects of Climate Change in the UK 2012: Current evidence, recommendations and research gaps.* Health Protection Agency, Centre for Radiation, Chemical and Environmental Hazards, UK. Available at: http://www.hpa.org.uk/webc/HPAwebFile/HPAweb_C/1317135969235 [Accessed 28 May 2013].

Vardoulakis, S., Solazzo, E., and Lumbreras, J. (2011). Intra-urban and street scale variability of BTEX, NO_2 and O_3 in Birmingham, UK: Implications for exposure assessment. *Atmospheric Environment,* **45**, 5069–5078.

World Health Organization (WHO) (2000). 2nd ed. *Air Quality Guidelines for Europe.* WHO Regional Publications, European Series, No. 91.

World Health Organization (WHO) (2006). *Air Quality Guidelines for Particulate Matter, Ozone, Nitrogen Dioxide and Sulphur Dioxide, Global update 2005, Summary of risk assessment.* Available at: http://www.euro.who.int/en/what-we-do/health-topics/environment-and-health/Housing-and-health/publications/pre-2009/air-quality-guidelines.-global-update-2005.-particulate-matter,-ozone,-nitrogen-dioxide-and-sulphur-dioxide [Accessed 10 April 2013].

World Health Organization (WHO) (2008). *World Health Statistics 2008.* Available at: http://www.who.int/gard/news_events/World_Health_Statistics_2008/en/ [accessed 10 April 2013].

World Health Organization (WHO) (2011). *Asthma Factsheet No 203, May 2011.* Available at: http://www.who.int/mediacentre/factsheets/fs307/en/index.html [accessed 1 April 2013].

World Health Organization (WHO) Regional Office for Europe (2001). *Quantification of the Health Effects of Exposure to Air Pollution: Report of a WHO Working Group, Bilthoven, Netherlands, 20–22 November 2000.* Available at: http://www.euro.who.int/en/health-topics/environment-and-health/air-quality/publications/pre2009/quantification-of-health-effects-of-exposure-to-air-pollution [Accessed 10 April 2013].

World Health Organization (WHO) Regional Office for Europe (2010). *WHO Guidelines for Indoor Air Quality: Selected pollutants.* Available at: http://www.euro.who.int/en/publications/abstracts/who-guidelines-for-indoor-air-quality-selected-pollutants [Accessed 10 April 2013].

Chapter 5

Water and public health

Gary Lau, Stephen Robjohns, Frances Pollitt, Meera Cush, and Britta Gadeberg

Learning objectives

By the end of this chapter the reader will be able to:
- understand the importance of wholesome water to public health
- understand the main European and UK water quality legislative frameworks and the roles and responsibilities of the regulators
- understand the different types of water supplies, common chemical contaminants, and their associated public health implications
- understand the basic principles of water supplies and discharges, and waste water treatments
- understand how health-based standards and guidelines are developed and their application to public health
- understand the approach used to investigate and risk assess water-related chemical incidents through case studies.

Introduction

The United Nations General Assembly declared that access to safe and clean drinking water and sanitation are essential to health and a key component of effective policy for health protection. The World Health Organization (WHO) defines safe drinking water as that required for all usual domestic purposes (including drinking, food preparation, and personal hygiene), which does not present any significant health risk over a lifetime of consumption and takes into account different sensitivities that may occur between life stages (WHO, 2011a).

It has been apparent that, in some WHO regions, investments of any scale in water supply and sanitation can benefit the economy by reducing associated adverse health effects and healthcare costs. This would outweigh the costs of undertaking the interventions. It is essential that countries develop and implement national drinking water quality standards, taking into account environmental, dietary, social, and other conditions that could affect potential exposure (WHO, 2011a).

The regulatory context in the UK

Drinking Water Inspectorate

The Drinking Water Inspectorate (DWI), formed in 1990 on the privatisation of the water industry, is the drinking water quality regulator for England and Wales and is part of the Department for Environment, Food and Rural Affairs (Defra). The DWI acts independently of government and its Chief Inspector is appointed by the Secretary of State for Environment, Food and Rural Affairs (in England) and the National Assembly for Wales.

The overarching objective of the DWI is to maintain public confidence in the safety and quality of public water supplies, which is achieved through the exercise of its powers of reporting, audit, inspection, enforcement, and prosecution. Additionally, the DWI has a role in providing government with advice on water supply and quality matters.

The Water Industry Act 1991 (the 1991 Act), amended by the Water Act 2003 (the 2003 Act), sets out the regulatory framework for water supplies in England and Wales, which defines the powers and duties under which DWI operates and also the duties of water companies and licensees. The Secretary of State for Environment, Food and Rural Affairs (in England) and the National Assembly for Wales are the authorities responsible for regulating the quality of public supplies under the 1991 Act (DWI, 2009).

A non-legally binding Memorandum of Understanding (MOU) sets out the agreed framework for cooperation between national regulators in the area of drinking management and regulations. The MOU is between the Environment Agency (EA) and the United Kingdom Drinking Water Regulators: DWI for England and Wales, the Drinking Water Quality Regulator for Scotland (DWQR), and the Drinking Water Inspectorate for Northern Ireland (DWINI) (DWI, 2010).

DWINI regulates drinking water quality in Northern Ireland for public and private supplies under a MOU between the Department of Regional Development and the Department of the Environment. It is a unit of the Northern Ireland Environment Agency (NIEA). Its enforcement powers are contained within the Water Supply (Water Quality) Regulations (Northern Ireland) 2007/147 (as amended), the Water Supply (Domestic Distribution Systems) Regulations (Northern Ireland) 2010/157, and the Private Water Supplies Regulations (Northern Ireland) 2009/413 (as amended).

The primary legislation pertaining to water supplies in Scotland is the Water (Scotland) Act 1980. The Drinking Water Quality Regulator for Scotland (DWQR), an independent regulator, is responsible for enforcing the Water Supply (Water Quality) (Scotland) Regulations 2001; the regulations relating to the quality of water supplied by Scottish Water are the Water Supply (Water Quality) (Scotland) Regulations 2001.

Wholesome water

Many of the standards come from the 1998 European Drinking Water Directive, often based on the WHO Guidelines for drinking-water quality, which came into force on 25 December 2003 (DWI, 2009). The Directive focuses on those parameters of importance to human health and others that relate to the control of water treatment processes and the aesthetic quality of drinking water. Member states are allowed to set additional or tighter national standards to secure the good quality of drinking water already achieved and to prevent it from deteriorating in the future (DWI, 2009).

Drinking water must be wholesome at the time of supply under the 1991 Act. Wholesomeness is defined by reference to drinking water quality standards and other requirements set out in the Water Supply (Water Quality) Regulations 2000 (as amended) for England and the Water Supply (Water Quality) Regulations 2001 (as amended) for Wales.

Public water supplies

A public water supply is defined as one provided for the purposes of drinking, washing, cooking, or food production by a statutorily appointed water company under the 1991 Act. A licence can also be granted to a water company to supply water in part of another water company's supply area. This is known as an 'inset appointment'. Non-domestic customers who use at least 50 megalitres (Ml) per year of water in a set of premises are able to purchase water from either their existing water company or from a licensed water supplier under the 2003 Act (DWI, 2009).

There are two kinds of licence: a retail water supply licence (the holder can buy and sell water) and a combined licence (the holder can introduce its own source of water into the network, as well as buying and selling water). The quality of water resources (groundwater, rivers, streams, lakes, raw water reservoirs) is regulated by the EA in England, a non-departmental public body of the Department for Environment, Food and Rural Affairs (DWI, 2009). Established on 1 April 2013, Natural Resources Wales is now responsible for managing water resources and improving water quality within Wales.

Private water supplies

Private water supplies as defined by the 1991 Act are those that are not provided by statutorily appointed water companies. They are highly variable in terms of their size and specific circumstances. Private water supplies are usually found in rural or remote areas of the countryside, but they are also occasionally used in the manufacture of certain foods and beverages and may serve various public buildings such as hospitals and hotels or, more commonly, campsites and leisure parks.

In England and Wales, the quality of private water supplies is the responsibility of local authorities through the implementation of the Private Water Supplies Regulations in 2009 (England) and 2010 (Wales). The drinking water standards applicable to private supplies are the same as those for public supplies, but for the smallest public supplies much more emphasis is placed on risk assessment and risk mitigation rather than very occasional monitoring. The role of DWI in respect of private supplies is to provide expert technical advice to local authorities, ensuring consistency of interpretation of drinking water legislation (DWI, 2009).

The DWI is responsible for collecting information from local authorities and publishing public reports annually, including information about public water supplies. For the majority of public health professionals, the provision of health protection advice to a local authority in respect of a private water supply is their most common area of work in relation to drinking water (DWI, 2009).

In Scotland, DWQR reports on the quality of private water supplies and provides guidance to local authorities who regulate them under the Private Water Supply (Scotland) Regulations 2006.

Fresh, marine, surface, and underground water

The EA in England and NRW in Wales are responsible for maintaining or improving the quality of fresh, marine, surface, and underground water. They have a duty to secure the proper use of water resources and monitor water in the environment, and to issue 'abstraction licences' to regulate who can take water from the environment (EA, 2012a). The European Water Framework Directive, which came into force on 22 December 2000, allows them to plan and deliver a better water environment, focussing on ecology. The Directive will help to protect and enhance the quality of:

- surface freshwater (including lakes, streams, and rivers)
- groundwater
- groundwater-dependent ecosystems
- estuaries
- coastal waters out to one nautical mile (EA, 2012b).

As the environmental regulator for the water industry in England, the EA informs and advises on the water industry's environmental performance in the delivery of existing environmental requirements by:

- monitoring compliance with their consents
- recording the number of pollution incidents
- taking and monitoring enforcement action (EA, 2012a).

The EA has developed a long-term strategy for water resources for the next 25 years, which considers the needs of both the environment and society (EA, 2012a).

The Water Management Unit (WMU) is a unit within the Northern Ireland Environment Agency (NIEA) responsible for protecting the aquatic environment under the Water (Northern Ireland) Order 1999. It has a duty to promote the conservation of the water resources and the cleanliness of water in waterways and underground, including the control of effluent discharges. In Scotland, the Scottish Environment Protection Agency (SEPA) is the responsible body for these functions.

Common sources of chemical pollutants and their associated public health implications

Drinking water is commonly sourced from either surface water or groundwater. Generally, groundwater requires less treatment than surface water. However, once a groundwater supply becomes contaminated it is very difficult to remediate and often no longer usable. Supplies from various sources may be blended before being put in the distribution system, as water from different sources will have different compositions (i.e. mineral and organic contents). In addition, some minerals are naturally present in water due to geology as opposed to anthropogenic sources. A selection of chemical contaminants that can be found in water supplies and their potential effects on health are described in the following sections.

Aluminium

Aluminium is the most abundant metal in the Earth's crust. Aluminium occurs naturally in soil, water, and air in the form of silicates, oxides, and hydroxides. Aluminium salts are widely used in water treatment as coagulants to reduce organic matter, colour, turbidity, and microorganism levels. Such use may lead to increased concentrations of aluminium in water. Other sources of aluminium for the general population are foods, particularly those containing aluminium compounds used as food additives, and aluminium-containing medicines. The contribution of drinking water to the total oral exposure to aluminium is usually less than 5 per cent of the total intake (WHO, 2010).

Cases of dialysis encephalopathy have been reported in patients with renal impairment as a result of intravenous administration of dialysis fluids containing high levels of aluminium. This is a degenerative neurological syndrome characterised by the gradual loss of motor, speech, and cognitive functions (IPCS, 1997). Aluminium has been proposed to play a role in the development of Alzheimer's disease, but the data are conflicting. Aluminium-containing over-the-counter products, such as antacids and buffered aspirin, are considered safe in healthy individuals at recommended doses based on historical use (HPA, 2012a; WHO, 2003a; WHO, 2010).

Those groups most susceptible to aluminium exposure are those with impaired renal function, because this can elevate aluminium concentrations in the body, and haemodialysis patients receiving tap water by intravascular administration in the home (IPCS, 1997).

Arsenic

Arsenic is a metalloid element that occurs naturally in soil and can dissolve in ground water. Some areas of the world have very high natural levels of arsenic and adverse health effects have been associated with consuming water in these regions (HPA, 2011). Coagulation using either aluminium or ferric salts can remove a high proportion, at least, of arsenic (V) (IPCS, 1981a).

Health effects resulting from arsenic exposure include skin lesions, peripheral vascular disease, peripheral neuropathy, and an increased risk of cancer of the skin, bladder, and lung (HPA, 2011; WHO, 2011b). Epidemiological studies of the rates of specific cancers in people consuming high levels of arsenic in drinking water, typically in excess of 300 µg/l, were used by the WHO to estimate the risk posed by exposure to arsenic below 50 µg/l. Nevertheless, there is still considerable uncertainty as to the actual level of risk associated with the consumption of drinking water containing arsenic below 50 µg/l and it is not possible to identify a level of exposure that is completely free from risk. Therefore, exposure to arsenic should be as low as reasonably practicable. This is why the WHO lowered the drinking water guideline value from 50 µg/l to 10 µg/l, since this was considered to be a practicable, technically achievable limit (HPA, 2011; WHO, 2011b).

Boron

Boron is a widely occurring element in minerals found in the Earth's crust. The majority of boron resides in the ocean and major world deposits are found in Turkey, the USA, Argentina, Russia, Chile, China, and Peru (IPCS, 1998a). Boron compounds are used in the manufacture of glass, soaps, and detergents, and as flame retardants. Naturally occurring boron is present in groundwater primarily as a result of leaching from rocks and soils containing borates and borosilicates. The borate content of surface water can be increased as a result of wastewater discharges, but this use has decreased significantly, and levels of boron in wastewater discharges continue to fall. There are conflicting views on whether boron is an essential nutrient for humans (WHO, 2009).

Human exposure to large amounts of boron over short periods of time have been reported to cause mainly gastrointestinal disturbances such as nausea and diarrhoea. Other effects reported include body hair loss, skin lesions, seizure disorders, fever, and general malaise. The estimated lethal dose ranges between 3000–6000 mg in infants and 15,000–20,000 mg in adults. Repeated oral exposures to boric acid or borax in laboratory animals have demonstrated that the reproductive system and developing fetus are the most sensitive targets of boron toxicity. The main effects reported are testicular lesions in male animals, and decreased viability and an increased rate of congenital anomalies in the fetuses of pregnant animals (WHO, 2009).

Copper

Copper is an essential nutrient (FSA, 2003; WHO, 2004a). Sources of copper intake include food, drinking water, supplements, and prescribed medicines. The taste of copper in drinking water has been described as metallic, bitter, and persistent (IPCS, 1998b). Copper is used to make pipes, valves, and fittings and is present in alloys and coatings. The primary source in drinking water is the corrosion of copper plumbing materials within houses and concentrations vary widely (WHO, 2004a). In some cases, drinking water may make a substantial additional contribution to the total daily intake of copper, particularly in households where corrosive waters have stood in copper pipes (IPCS, 1998b).

Concentrations of copper greater than 5 mg/l may render water unpalatable, although individuals can adapt to such levels. Aesthetic considerations relating to copper levels in drinking water include blue or green staining of plumbing fixtures, hair, and laundry (IPCS, 1998b). Acute copper toxicity is rare because, in high quantities, it induces vomiting and has an unpleasant taste. Signs of toxicity include salivation, abdominal pain, nausea, vomiting, and diarrhoea (similar to symptoms of food poisoning). Vomiting has been associated with consumption of beverages contaminated with copper ranging from 25–840 mg/l. Ingestion of large amounts of copper sulfate (in excess of 100 g) may cause intravascular haemolysis (breakdown of red blood cells), acute liver failure, acute kidney failure, shock, coma, or death (FSA, 2003).

There are limited data on the effects of chronic exposure to copper in humans (FSA, 2003). Chronic systemic toxicity is rare because the amount in the body is controlled by homeostatic mechanisms. In the general human population, the key adverse effects usually associated with excess copper intake are gastrointestinal, as described previously (FSA, 2003; WHO, 2004a).

Patients on haemodialysis receiving tap water by intravascular administration at home and people with chronic liver disease are potentially sensitive to copper excess. Children may be at increased risk of copper toxicity due to a combination of more efficient uptake and immature biliary excretion (FSA, 2003). However, copper accumulates naturally in the fetus during the third trimester of pregnancy without apparent adverse effects, suggesting that newborn babies may be resistant to high levels of hepatic copper. Groups who are susceptible to adverse effects of copper are those with genetic defects in the homeostatic control mechanisms, such as sufferers of Wilson's disease (failure of normal copper excretion into the bile and of incorporation into ceruloplasmin) and idiopathic copper toxicosis (ICT, characterised by accumulation of copper in the liver) (FSA, 2003; WHO, 2004a).

Iron

Iron is one of the most abundant metals in the Earth's crust and is found naturally in surface and groundwater. Iron may also be present in drinking water as a result of corrosion of iron pipes or use of iron coagulants (WHO, 2003b). Iron is an essential element in human nutrition and, in general, the human body regulates the level of iron by controlling the amount absorbed from food and drink, according to iron status. Adults have often taken iron supplements for extended periods without deleterious effects and the WHO considers that an intake of 400–1000 µg/kg bw/day is unlikely to cause adverse effects in healthy people (JECFA, 1983; WHO, 2003b).

Although adverse effects from consumption of drinking water containing iron are unlikely in healthy individuals, some adverse effects have been reported following high levels of iron consumption (for example, as the result of excessive supplement ingestion). Potential adverse effects are largely gastrointestinal; constipation is most common but nausea, diarrhoea, and vomiting can also occur. Chronic ingestion of excessive iron may result in tissue damage, including cirrhosis of the liver and impaired heart and endocrine function (FSA, 2003; JECFA, 1983).

Individuals with metabolic defects that impair the ability to regulate iron in the body, such as hereditary haemochromatosis (inability to regulate iron absorption and distribution), β-thalassaemia (inability to create red blood cells), and sideroblastic anaemia (inability of red blood cells to incorporate iron) are at higher risk from excessive exposure to iron. Individuals with pre-existing gastrointestinal tract disease or chronic hepatitis have also been shown to be vulnerable to the toxic effects of iron (FSA, 2003; JECFA, 1983; WHO, 2003b).

Lead

Lead is a naturally occurring element in the Earth's crust. Lead has historically been widely used in plumbing, and also in paint and in leaded petrol. Human exposure to lead occurs principally via food and drinking water. Lead is rarely naturally present in raw water sources; rather, it comes primarily from plumbing systems containing lead in pipes, solder, and fittings. Before 1970, many smaller water pipes were made from lead; however, lead pipes have not been permitted for this purpose since then. Therefore, lead plumbing is found in older properties and longstanding private supplies, and may be present at any point from source to tap, including linings for holding tanks (HPA, 2012a). In hard water areas, the scale formed inside the pipes protects the water from the lead. In soft water areas, there is a greater likelihood of lead from pipes being present in the water (DWI, 2010). Lead-based solder may be another, albeit uncommon, source of lead in water, although its use to join copper water piping is no longer allowed. However, it may be mistakenly used by unqualified plumbers as it is still sold for use on closed central heating systems.

High levels of short-term exposure can cause nausea, vomiting, diarrhoea, or kidney damage (HPA, 2012b; IARC, 2006). Lead can accumulate in the body, particularly in the skeleton (HPA, 2012b; WHO, 2011c). If exposure to relatively high levels of lead continues for a long time, people may become anaemic, lethargic, and irritable or show other symptoms such as headache, muscle tremors, kidney or liver damage, nausea, vomiting, or high blood pressure. Long-term exposure to high levels can also affect male and female reproduction (HPA, 2012b; IARC, 2006). Children with high amounts of lead in their bones may have delayed growth (HPA, 2012b; IARC, 2006; WHO, 2011c).

The most important adverse effect of lead following long-term, low level exposure is on intellectual and cognitive development in children, although there is also a risk of increased blood pressure and kidney toxicity in adults (HPA, 2012b; WHO, 2011a; WHO, 2011c). It has not been possible to identify a threshold for these critical effects (CONTAM, 2010). Therefore, current advice is that exposure to lead should be as low as reasonably practicable.

The fetus, infants, and children up to 6 years of age are particularly sensitive to lead. Children exposed to lead when in the womb or during the first few years of life may have a lower IQ, behavioural problems, or nerve damage (HPA, 2012b; JECFA, 2010; WHO, 2011a; WHO, 2011c).

Manganese

Manganese is one of the most abundant metals in the Earth's crust and usually occurs with iron. Manganese is naturally occurring in many surface water and groundwater sources, particularly in anaerobic or low oxidation conditions, and this is the most likely source of manganese in drinking water (WHO, 2011d).

The greatest exposure to manganese is usually from food. Manganese is an essential element for humans and adverse effects can result from both deficiency and overexposure. The mean levels of manganese in drinking water are usually about 5–25 µg/l, but individual samples from municipal supplies have shown concentrations ranging from trace levels to 100 μg/l (IPCS, 1981b). Reports of individuals exposed to high doses of manganese (for example as the result of consuming excessive mineral supplements) have described neurological impairment, including fatigue, muscle pain, tremor, and impaired reflexes (FSA, 2003; WHO, 2011d).

A few epidemiological studies report adverse neurological effects following extended exposure to high levels in drinking water, but there are a number of problems in interpreting these studies (FSA, 2003; WHO, 2011d). A recent Canadian study suggested that consumption of manganese from untreated groundwater (mean concentration 34 μg/l, range 1–2700 μg/l) was associated with intellectual impairment in children (Bouchard et al., 2010). However, the manganese in this study may have been more bioavailable than manganese in treated UK supplies and other studies have failed to observe adverse effects following exposure from drinking water (HPA, 2012a).

Individuals with anaemia may be vulnerable to the toxic effects of manganese due to the increased absorption that occurs in states of iron deficiency. Other vulnerable subgroups are those individuals with impaired biliary clearance or impaired or immature manganese homeostasis, such as patients with liver disease, the elderly, and infants. It has also been reported that alcohol consumption and long-term use of anti-psychotic drugs increases the susceptibility of humans to manganese toxicity (FSA, 2003).

Nitrate and nitrite

Nitrate is an anion of nitrogen and oxygen, which is naturally present in the environment. It is produced during the natural decay of vegetable matter in soil or may be added as a fertiliser to arable land. Commercially, it is mainly used in inorganic fertilisers, but is also used in the production of explosives. The nitrate ion (NO_3^-) occurs naturally in drinking water as part of the nitrogen cycle (IARC, 2010; WHO, 2011a). Rainfall washes nitrate from the subsoil into ground and surface water and may give rise to elevated concentrations in drinking water. However, nitrate can also reach surface waters and groundwater as a result of agricultural activity, from wastewater treatment, and from oxidation of nitrogenous waste products in human and animal excreta, including septic tanks (IARC, 2010; JECFA, 2002; WHO, 2011a). The nitrite ion (NO_2^-) is also naturally present in the environment and drinking water. It can be formed by the reduction of the nitrate ion. Nitrite can also be formed by bacteria during stagnation of nitrate-containing and oxygen-poor drinking water in galvanised steel pipes, or during poorly controlled residual disinfection using chloramination (WHO, 2011a).

Ingested nitrate can be converted to nitrite in the gastrointestinal tract. Nitrite is involved in the oxidation of haemoglobin to methaemoglobin (MetHb) resulting in a condition known as methaemoglobinaemia (a reduced ability of red blood cells to transport oxygen to tissues). This condition occurs more readily in bottle-fed babies and is then known as infantile methaemoglobinaemia (IM), also known as 'blue baby syndrome'. Clinical symptoms of mild IM include cyanosis (bluish discolouration) of the skin, lips, tongue, and nose, fatigue, and dizziness. There is good evidence to suggest that the risk of methaemoglobinaemia is increased in the presence of simultaneous gastrointestinal infections, as endogenous nitrate formation is increased, and thus the reduction of nitrate to nitrite increases. Water intake during such infections may also rise to combat dehydration, therefore adding to the nitrate burden. Methaemoglobinaemia has most frequently been associated with private wells, which have a high probability of microbial contamination (IARC, 2010; JECFA, 2002; WHO, 2011a).

It has been suggested that pregnant women may be more susceptible to methaemoglobinaemia, but there is minimal evidence to support this from exposure to nitrate in drinking water (Manassaram et al., 2010). Individuals deficient in the enzymes glucose-6-phosphate dehydrogenase or MetHb reductase may be more susceptible to methaemoglobinaemia (IARC, 2010; WHO, 2011a).

It has been proposed that there is an increased risk of gastric cancer under conditions of low gastric acidity, which could be associated with the endogenous formation of potentially carcinogenic N-nitroso compounds. Also, high levels of N-nitroso compounds, as well as high nitrate levels, have been found in the gastric juice of achlorhydric (low levels of stomach acid) patients. Consequently, it has been hypothesised that such patients could be considered as a special risk group for gastric cancer and it is plausible that other groups of individuals with low gastric acidity, such as those using proton pump inhibitors or antacids, could also have an increased risk of gastric cancer. However, overall, the epidemiology data provide no convincing evidence to support an association between exposure to nitrate in drinking water and cancer (including gastric cancer) (HPA, 2012a; IARC, 2010; JECFA, 2002; WHO, 2011a).

Pesticides

Pesticides are chemical compounds used to kill pests, including insects, rodents, fungi, and unwanted plants (weeds). Pesticides are used in public health to kill vectors of disease, such as mosquitoes, and in agriculture to kill pests that damage crops. By their nature, pesticides are potentially toxic to other organisms, including humans, and need to be used and disposed of safely. Non-occupational human exposure to pesticides occurs principally via food. Pesticides may be present in source waters (particularly surface water-derived supplies) from the natural run-off from farms and other land where pesticides have been employed (HPA, 2012a).

Aldrin and dieldrin are highly effective pesticides for soil-dwelling pests and for the protection of wooden structures against termites and wood borers (WHO, 2003c). Dieldrin has also been used against insects of public health importance. Although the use of aldrin and dieldrin has been severely restricted or banned in many parts of the world since the early 1970s for environmental reasons, the pesticides are still used in termite control in some countries (ATSDR, 2002; WHO, 2003c; WHO, 2011a). Both aldrin and dieldrin are banned in the UK and the rest of the EU. These pesticides are rarely present in groundwater, as little leaching from soils occurs (ATSDR, 2002; WHO, 2003c).

Aldrin decomposes to dieldrin and is stored as dieldrin in body tissues. Its chronic toxicity is related to the level of dieldrin in the body. Both aldrin and dieldrin are highly toxic to humans, the target organs being the central nervous system, kidneys, and liver. However, most of those poisoned by aldrin or dieldrin recover, and irreversible effects have not been reported (ATSDR, 2002; WHO, 2003c). The lethal dose of dieldrin is estimated to be approximately 10 mg/kg bw/day (WHO, 2003c). Toxic exposures to aldrin produce neurological and gastrointestinal effects. Haemolytic anaemia has also been reported following oral exposure to aldrin and dieldrin, but this is likely to be rare. The International Agency for Research on Cancer (IARC) has categorised aldrin and dieldrin as Group 3 chemicals (unclassifiable as to human carcinogenic potential) (ATSDR, 2002; WHO, 2003c; WHO, 2011a).

Clopyralid is a pyridine herbicide used to kill unwanted annual and perennial broadleaf plants in turf and lawn, range, pasture, right-of-ways, and some agricultural crops. Clopyralid is not metabolised in humans, but it is widely distributed in the body, with the highest concentration found in the liver. There is no evidence that clopyralid accumulates in the body. No groups are known to be particularly susceptible to the toxicity of clopyralid. There are limited data available on the adverse effects of clopyralid in humans. It is a severe eye irritant and repeated or prolonged dermal contact with clopyralid may cause mild skin irritation (HPA, 2009).

Metaldehyde is used primarily as a molluscicide bait for controlling slugs and snails. Metaldehyde is toxic following ingestion, skin contact, or, to a lesser extent, inhalation. There have been several reports of human poisoning by metaldehyde. The initial signs and symptoms of acute metaldehyde toxicity usually occur 1–3 hours after ingestion and include salivation, facial flushing, nausea, vomiting, abdominal pain, accelerated heart rate (tachycardia), and drowsiness. Higher doses of metaldehyde may cause rigid muscles and spasms, tremor, seizures, coma, and death (HPA, 2008).

Selenium

Selenium is present in the Earth's crust and is found naturally in groundwater and surface water. Surface waters seem much less likely to contain excessive levels of selenium than groundwater (IPCS, 1986). Drinking water rarely contributes much selenium to a person's total daily intake; foodstuffs constitute the main source of selenium for the general population (IPCS, 1986; WHO, 2011a). Selenium is an essential trace element in human nutrition and it is incorporated into proteins (WHO, 2004b; WHO, 2011a).

Early agricultural uses of selenium compounds as pesticides were very limited and short-lived. Later use of selenium compounds as feed additives or injectables for the prevention of selenium deficiency diseases in farm animals represented a source for environmental contamination, but compared with the levels already present in most feeds and the amounts found in soils, even in the deficient areas, this source seemed insignificant (IPCS, 1986).

Acute high oral doses of selenite and other selenium compounds can cause symptoms such as nausea, diarrhoea, abdominal pain, chills, tremor, numbness in limbs, irregular menstrual bleeding, marked hair loss, and neurological disturbance (restlessness, spasms, and tachycardia). Chronic high dietary intakes of selenium have resulted in gastrointestinal disturbances, skin discolouration, tooth decay, and neurological effects. Convulsions and paralysis may then develop, corresponding with high urinary selenium levels. Long-term selenium exposure can also manifest in effects on the liver, such as decreased prothrombin (a blood-clotting chemical) synthesis. Selenium toxicity is cumulative and no susceptible groups have been identified (HPA, 2012a).

Disinfection by-products

Disinfection of drinking water supplies is essential for the prevention of infectious waterborne diseases. Disinfection may result in the formation of a number of disinfection by-products (DBPs) due to the reaction of the disinfectants with naturally occurring organic and inorganic substances in the source water (Krasner, 2009). Chlorination is the main disinfection process used in the UK and trihalomethanes (THMs) and haloacetic acids (HAAs) are the main DBPs formed. Haloacetonitriles (HANs), halophenols, haloaldehydes, and haloketones can also be formed (COT, 2008).

THMs (typically bromoform, bromodichloromethane, chloroform, and dibromochloromethane) are not usually found in unpolluted raw water sources, but are generally present in chlorinated or treated water; concentrations are generally less than 100 µg/l, with chloroform being the dominant compound in most cases (WHO, 2011a). DBPs are formed through complex reactions of a chemical disinfectant with an organic precursor, such as the natural organic matter (NOM). The disinfectants can oxidise a complex NOM molecule into simpler moieties, which are then reactive with other chemicals or the residual disinfectant (Krasner, 2009).

THMs can cause taste or odour issues in drinking water (Scottish Executive, 2006) but are not usually expected to cause acute adverse health effects. The main focus of concern with regard to adverse health effects of THMs in drinking water has been potential carcinogenicity and adverse developmental or reproductive effects (Krasner, 2009).

IARC has not classified chlorinated drinking water as to its carcinogenicity to humans (Group 3); however, chloroform and bromodichloromethane have been classified as possibly carcinogenic to humans (Group 2B). The UK committee on carcinogenicity of chemicals in food consumer products and the environment (COC) reviewed the available evidence on cancer and chlorinated drinking water and concluded that the evidence for a causal association between cancer and exposure to DBPs is limited and any such association is unlikely to be strong (COC, 2008).

The UK committee on toxicity of chemicals in food consumer products and the environment (COT) reviewed the available evidence and concluded that in human studies there is no consistent relationship between chlorinated drinking water and adverse pregnancy outcomes, including low birth weight, pregnancy loss, pre-term delivery, and congenital malformations (COT, 2008).

Careful management of the treatment processes and disinfection can control the formation of DBPs. Typically THM formation can be controlled by:

- reducing organic content of the raw water before disinfection, for example using granular activated carbon (GAC)

- modifying disinfection practice or use of disinfectants other than chlorine; however, the use of disinfectants such as chlorine dioxide or ozone may simply result in the creation of alternative DBPs (Krasner, 2009).

Although efforts should be made to minimise the formation of DBPs this should not compromise the effective disinfection of drinking water (COC, 2008).

Drinking water sources and treatment

There is a wide range of treatment processes that can be used to produce water that is safe to drink and aesthetically pleasing. The actual processes selected will depend on the nature of the raw water source and the intended use of the treated water (Binnie and Kimber, 2009). The two principal raw water sources are groundwater and surface water. Depending on the hydrogeology of a basin, the levels of human activity in the vicinity of the source, and other factors, a wide range of water qualities can be encountered. Surface waters typically have higher concentrations of particulate matter than groundwater and groundwater has increased concentrations of dissolved minerals due to the long contact times between subsurface water with rocks and minerals (Crittenden et al., 2012). Conventional water treatment usually consists of some or all of the following main processes:

- Coagulation and flocculation: to remove smaller particles and microbes. Chemicals are added to promote the formation of agglomerates, trapping impurities in the process, so that they can then be removed from the surface of the water.
- Filtration: to remove particles, organic matter, and microbes. This is usually done by using sand filters; either slow or rapid sand filtration or a combination of the two.
- GAC: to remove organic substances, in particular pesticides, and to eliminate taste and odour problems. Chemicals are removed from the water through carbon adsorption. The use of GAC is widespread but is not used in all water treatment works (WTWs).
- Disinfection: to kill any remaining microbes and to ensure that water remains of high microbiological quality in the distribution system. Chlorination is the most widely used disinfection method, achieved by using free chlorine, chlorine dioxide, or chloramines. Ozonation and/or treatment with UV radiation can also be used.
- pH adjustment: to correct for acidity or alkalinity. Some waters require the addition of chemicals to adjust the pH to prevent corrosion of pipes and fittings in the distribution system.

Additional treatment methods may be used if particular contaminants are a problem, for example membrane filtration may be used to combat cryptosporidium, a parasite that causes enteritis. Orthophosphorous acid or sodium phosphate compounds are added to some supplies to reduce plumbosolvency, the dissolution of lead from old water pipes.

Wastewater treatment and disposal

Wastewater may include domestic, municipal, or industrial liquid waste products, which are usually carried by a sewerage network and treated before discharge or disposal. There is also storm water from precipitation run-off and infiltration/inflow, where extraneous water enters the sewerage system from the ground by various means. Sewers can be classified into three groups, depending on the type of wastewater they carry:

- Foul sewers: these carry sewage and trade effluent, which require treatment before discharge.
- Surface sewers or drains: these carry away rainwater run-off from roads and hard-covered areas. The water is usually relatively clean and can therefore be discharged directly to a watercourse, although there may be contamination from vehicle fuels or spills.
- Combined sewers: these carry away a combination of wastewater and rainwater run-off. They can also function as storm drains in periods of heavy rain when large quantities of water need to be discharged.

A sewerage network is the physical infrastructure that conveys sewage from its origin to the point of eventual treatment, i.e. a WWTW, in order to produce an environmentally safe fluid waste stream and a solid waste/treated sludge suitable for disposal or reuse, for example in fertilisers. Conventional wastewater treatment consists of some or all of the following main processes:

- Pre-treatment: to remove large floating materials before treatment and to protect downstream mechanical equipment. Grit channels remove grit after screening, in order to reduce abrasion of equipment and settlement in the biological treatment plant. Equalisation is carried out to equalise flow rates or to dilute high concentrations of effluents.
- Primary treatment: to settle wastewater, separating it into a clarified effluent and liquid/solid sludge (primary sludge). The objective is to produce an effluent with improved quality for the next treatment stage. Primary treatment can be chemically enhanced by the addition of coagulants, for example alum, iron salts, or lime, to promote flocculation of fine suspended particles, enabling them to be removed more easily.
- Secondary treatment: to biodegrade organic compounds in the effluent and to reduce the level of nutrients, specifically nitrogen and phosphorous, which are capable of causing eutrophication (excess of nutrients) of the waters into which the treated wastewater is discharged.

In the UK, most liquid discharges from WWTWs are classified as trade effluent. Therefore, where the discharge is to controlled water as defined in national legislation, consent is required from the regulators (Binnie and Kimber, 2009).

Sludge treatment and disposal

All biological processes generate sludge, and some produce twice the mass of solids that is present in the untreated wastewater. Up to 50 per cent of crude sewage solids may be inorganic. The sludge produced by a WWTW is typically derived from the following sources:

- suspended solids in the raw water
- colour that is removed during treatment

- coagulants added during the process and any dissolved chemicals and hardness that precipitate out during treatment and softening
- other chemicals added during treatment such as polymers and bentonite
- biological growth within the processes (Binnie and Kimber, 2009).

With very few exceptions, most treatment technologies generate sludge, or several different types of sludge, which often have different characteristics and require separate treatment:

- Inorganic sludges: these represent waste of raw materials from separation processes and the material should always be recovered where possible. The basic properties of inorganic sludge are that it is inert, settles quickly, and forms a dense deposit.
- Organic sludges: these are frequently odorous and likely to undergo biological breakdown with release of noxious, flammable, and explosive gases. De-watering is usually difficult due to the biological bound water content. Untreated organic sludges represent a potential source of energy by digestion or incineration and a valuable soil conditioner/fertiliser.

The main objective of sludge treatment is to reduce the sludge's volume by reducing its water content. Conventional sludge treatment consists of some or all of the following main processes:

- Conditioning: sludge solids are treated with chemicals, for example coagulants, or various other means, such as pH adjustment, to prepare the sludge for subsequent de-watering processes.
- Thickening: to reduce the volume of sludge by removing a portion of the liquid fraction, typically using polymers.
- De-watering: this is a physical unit process used principally for the reduction of the moisture content of the sludge.
- Stabilisation: to reduce pathogens, eliminate offensive odours, and inhibit, reduce, or eliminate the potential for putrefaction.
- Composting: to stabilise organic wastes and produce humus (compost) through an aerobic bacterial decomposition process. Compost contains nutrients and organic carbon, which are excellent soil conditioners.

Final disposal of sludge and solids from treatment facilities is usually by one or more of the following methods:

- ocean dumping
- land spreading
- lagooning
- landfilling
- incineration.

Wastes that are disposed of to a landfill are classified as industrial waste. In England and Wales, they fall under the requirements of Part II of the Environmental Protection Act

1990, and the Waste Management Licensing Regulations 2006. A waste management licence is needed for authorised disposal (Birnie and Kimber, 2009).

Public health risk assessment

The drinking water standards that are applied to private water supplies are the same as those for public water supplies. An up-to-date risk assessment is required to establish whether there is a significant risk of supplying drinking water that would constitute 'a potential danger to human health'. Apart from microbiological, chemical, and radiological hazards, regulatory risk assessments also cover other physical and organisational hazards, which may result in a failure of the water supply (no water) or consumers rejecting the water for aesthetic reasons (DWI, 2009).

It is a requirement of water companies and local authorities to communicate effectively about their risk assessments with key stakeholders, which means that public health professionals, including Public Health England (PHE), will be briefed on, and consulted about, each specific risk assessment for water supplies in their areas. Through these consultations, they have the opportunity to understand the local water supply arrangements, to raise questions, and to satisfy themselves that they fully take account of the public health needs of the local community (DWI, 2009).

Communications that are sent to consumers in areas where drinking water quality is affected by an incident typically consist of one of three types of warning message:

- boil before use for drinking and food preparation (BWA)
- do not use for drinking or cooking (DND)
- do not use for drinking, cooking, or washing (DNU).

A BWA notice causes inconvenience in the home and can be disruptive to certain businesses (food and drink retailers and manufacturers) and public buildings (healthcare premises), but the water industry has substantive experience of their practical aspects, which are manageable, and the public is familiar with the concept. By contrast, a DND notice poses a more significant challenge to a water supplier due to the need to make alternative provisions of water supplies for drinking and cooking. These logistical problems are magnified and further compounded in the case of a DNU notice because of the hygiene issues implicit in restricting the public's access to piped water for showering and bathing. Furthermore, the public is unfamiliar with water restrictions of this nature and on a large scale, and a far wider range of businesses will be affected (DWI, 2009).

It is recommended that DNU notices are reserved for use only in circumstances where there is unequivocal evidence of persistent contamination of the water supply with a substance at a level where short-term exposure is known to give rise to adverse health effects in an otherwise healthy population, and measures to restore the water supply to normal are likely to be protracted (weeks rather than hours or days). Generally, the type of circumstances when a DNU notice may be considered are: where there is a major chemical pollution incident that cannot be contained by the water supplier through stopping abstraction;

an incident at the treatment works; or where the contamination has entered the treated water distribution system and the extent of the contaminated water cannot quickly be identified and contained/removed (DWI, 2009).

Another relevant scenario would be where the contaminant cannot be detected by a change in appearance, taste, or smell of the water (meaning consumers would not be alerted to the problem and thus are unlikely to take avoiding action). In most water quality incidents, therefore, the choice of warning notice to issue is between a BWA and a DND. Where there has been a loss of supplies due to a failure of an asset, the water supplier will be able to access records of water fittings inspections and identify whether there are any premises in the affected area classified as high risk in terms of the potential to cause water contamination due to back flow or back siphonage. All high risk premises are routinely inspected and checked to ensure adequate back flow protection is in place (DWI, 2009).

A BWA notice is the most appropriate one to use in 'loss of supply' incidents. As with DNU notices, the use of a DND notice should be reserved for situations where short-term exposure to a chemical is likely to give rise to adverse health effects. The above guidance relates to the general public, and in any incident, it is always important to separately consider the need to issue specific and different advice for vulnerable or sensitive users (DWI, 2009).

Health-based standards and guidelines and their application to public health

Heath-based standards and guidelines are established to ensure effective health protection and improvement at all levels of national development. Standards and guidelines should form part of an overall public health policy and take into account the contribution of drinking water to overall exposure to hazardous chemicals. Standards and guidelines need to be realistic, measurable, based on scientific data, and relevant to local financial, technical, and institutional resources (WHO, 2011a).

Development of health-based standards and guidelines

Water quality standards and guidelines are the most common form of health-based targets. Standards and guidelines are generally established on the basis of international risk assessments of the health effects associated with exposure to the chemicals that may be found in drinking water. In addition, it is necessary to take into account a number of contributing factors such as environmental, social, cultural, economic, dietary, and other conditions affecting potential exposure, as well as the default assumptions that are used to derive the guideline values. National targets may differ appreciably from guideline values since exposure to chemicals through drinking water is typically minor in comparison with that from other sources such as food, consumer products, and air, with a few important exceptions, for example arsenic. It may be considered more appropriate to take action to prevent exposure to a chemical from sources other than drinking water, for example lead from solders and petrol.

Water quality standards and guidelines should be considered in order to determine appropriate water treatment requirements, where they are necessary. Water quality standards and guidelines should be established for those chemicals that, following rigorous assessment, have been determined to be of significant health concern or of concern for the acceptability of the drinking water to consumers (WHO, 2011a).

Calculating intakes from chemical exposure

Health-based standards and guidelines for chemical parameters are set using a precautionary approach, on the basis of a lifetime's consumption of water and taking into account exposure through routes other than drinking water, for example food. Just because a standard has been set for a substance does not mean that it is present in drinking water. Other substances may occur only in very specific or local circumstances, for example leaching from fixtures and fittings or pipework within a specific building's water system (HPA, 2012a).

Default intakes of chemicals in drinking water can be estimated by using the following assumptions:

- an adult weighs 60 kg and drinks 2 l of the water per day
- a child weighs 10 kg and drinks 1 l of the water per day
- a bottle-fed baby weighs 5 kg and drinks 0.75 l of the water per day.

The risk to health can be assessed by comparing the concentration of a chemical in drinking water with the WHO health-based guideline value (where they exist):

- If the concentration of the chemical in drinking water is lower than the WHO health-based guideline value, it is of very minimal health risk.
- If the concentration is above the WHO health-based guideline value, it is possible to calculate intake by conducting the following calculation and comparing the intake value to an identified acceptable daily intake (ADI), tolerable daily intake (TDI), or other parameters that may be used to set the WHO health-based guideline value:
- Intake in adults from drinking water (mg/kg bw/day) = (concentration of chemical (mg/l) × 2)/60
- Intake in children from drinking water (mg/kg bw/day) = (concentration of chemical (mg/l) × 1)/10
- Intake in bottle-fed babies (mg/kg bw/day) = (concentration of chemical (mg/l) × 0.75)/5

However, consideration should be given to how long the individual has been/will be exposed to the chemical and to the possible contribution of other sources of the chemical, such as food. For a short-term exposure (one week or less) it is usually unnecessary to take other sources of the chemical into account but for long-term exposures, the ADI/TDI or similar parameters should be compared with total intake from all sources (HPA, 2012a).

Case Studies 5.1, 5.2, and 5.3 illustrate risk assessments from public water supplies.

Case Study 5.1: Carbetamide contamination in drinking water

The Centre for Radiation, Chemical and Environmental Hazards (CRCE) of Public Health England was notified of an incident involving carbetamide contamination in drinking water from a public water supply. Carbetamide is used as a pesticide (herbicide) in the UK. Carbetamide is considered to have relatively low mammalian toxicity (EFSA, 2010).

Carbetamide was detected at the above levels at two separate WTWs, which abstracted directly from a surface water source, a local river. The water treatment process included ozonation and GAC for pesticide removal prior to supply to a large population.

No specific prescribed concentration or value exists for carbetamide in the UK drinking water regulations; however, the detected results were above the 0.1 ìg/l prescribed concentration for an individual pesticide (see Table 5.1). It was therefore necessary to undertake a toxicological risk assessment in order to ascertain the magnitude of the issue at hand in terms of any risks to human health.

Table 5.1 Test results of pre-treatment and post-treatment samples

Sample	Minimum (µg/l)	Maximum (µg/l)
Pre-treatment	–	1.8
Post-treatment	0.16	0.44

In 2010, the European Food Safety Authority (EFSA) concluded a peer-review of the risk assessment report on carbetamide and an acceptable daily intake (ADI) of 0.06 mg/kg bw/day (or 60 µg/kg bw/day) was set for carbetamide (EFSA, 2010). This ADI was used as the basis of the public health risk assessment based on the following assumptions:

- an adult weighs 60 kg and drinks 2 l of the water per day
- a child weighs 10 kg and drinks 1 l of the water per day
- a bottle-fed baby weighs 5 kg and drinks 0.75 l of the water per day.

The risk assessment considered the consequences for consumers' health assuming a worst case scenario of lifetime consumption of drinking water containing carbetamide at 0.44 µg/l, the highest level detected within the public supply.

The calculated intake for an adult would be 0.015 µg/kg bw/day, that for a child would be 0.045 µg/kg bw/day, and that for an infant would be 0.066 µg/kg bw/day. The calculated intakes of 0.015, 0.044 and 0.066 µg/kg bw/day in adults, children, and infants, respectively, were 1000-fold or more below the ADI of 60 µg/kg bw/day. Therefore, it was concluded that there was no reason to expect adverse health effects, even if exposure to these levels were relatively chronic.

However, it must be noted that the full range of levels detected by the water company at the WTWs did exceed the UK prescribed concentration of 0.1 µg/l for the presence of carbetamide in drinking water. Therefore, it was recommended that the water company rectify the problem as soon as possible to ensure conformity with the regulator's water quality standards.

Case Study 5.2: Lead contamination in drinking water

An incident involving lead contamination in drinking water within a specialist school for children (attended by 59 children aged between 2 and 11) with speech, language, and communication needs was reported to CRCE. One of the school buildings dating back to the post-war era was believed to contain lead pipes, which prompted the school to start using bottled water for cooking and drinking.

Subsequently, the school requested testing by the water company. Test results are shown in Table 5.2 for samples taken at the kitchen tap and tank-fed tap in a playroom, which some kitchen staff had previously used for cooking despite the school having labelled it unsuitable for such use. Post-flush, the results at the tank-fed tap had risen, which was probably due to standing water being drawn into the tank from internal lead pipes.

Table 5.2 Test results of samples taken at the kitchen tap and tank-fed tap in the playroom

Source	Pre-flush (µg/l)	Post-flush (µg/l)
Kitchen tap	42.20	8.68
Tank-fed tap	17.60	23.00

The water company had identified a lead service pipe connection to the building and arranged to have the communication pipe replaced. The school was advised by the water company to replace all lead pipes within the building, including the supply pipe, and to stop using the tank-fed tap in the playroom for cooking and drinking. In the meantime, prolonged flushing before use, for example 5 minutes, was advised at the kitchen tap in the mornings as the length of lead pipes were estimated to be 60 m.

Since the post-flush lead levels were below the UK prescribed concentration (25 µg/l) for lead in drinking water, complete removal of lead was possible once the lead service pipe and any lead-containing materials within the plumbing system were removed. Although no symptoms of lead poisoning had been reported, there were concerns over whether or not the school children, as well as staff members, had suffered from the potentially chronic lead exposure. Specialist toxicological consideration was given in terms of a risk assessment for lead; the approach employed was similar to that recommended by the European Food Safety Authority's Panel on Contaminants in the Food Chain for its assessment of dietary exposure to lead (CONTAM, 2010).

It was impossible to rule out a potential risk of nephrotoxicity in adults and developmental neurotoxicity in children, fetuses, and infants using worst-case exposure assumptions. However, there were other site-specific exposure factors that needed to be taken into account in order to come up with a realistic public health approach to the incident:

- Realistically it was unlikely that the water consumed or used in food preparation from either of the taps would be consistently high.
- Only one meal was taken at the school and given the daily attendance pattern, any lead exposure at the school via drinking water was likely to be transient and of limited duration rather than continuous exposure.
- Although no set use pattern was reported, water may have been drawn from the kitchen tap for other purposes apart from cooking and drinking, for example cleaning, which would help the flushing of lead within the plumbing system.

Based on the fact that none of the post-flush test results exceeded the UK prescribed concentration of 25 µg/l for lead in drinking water and that chronic lead exposure at the school was realistically unlikely, it was concluded that the risk of exposure was low. However, CRCE identified several follow-up actions to minimise potential ongoing exposures:

- Prolonged flushing should be continually practised until all lead pipes within the building and the supply pipe were replaced and subsequent testing by the water company showed satisfactory results.

- Test results were based on a one-off sampling. Further monitoring could prove consistency and verify the test results.
- Investigation to be carried out in other school buildings to identify possible drinking water supplies contaminated with lead and followed up with appropriate protective measures and remediation.
- Although no symptoms of lead poisoning had been reported, the situation was communicated to all families and staff members providing reassurance that it was unlikely to be detrimental to public health. In addition, they were recommended to seek clinical advice and information from either a GP or the NHS Direct hotline (NHS, 2012) if there were health concerns.

Case Study 5.3: Unusual tastes and odours in drinking water

An incident was reported to CRCE involving unusual tastes and odours in drinking water from a public water supply. Prior to the incident being reported, the water company had received an increasing number of taste and odour complaints from customers, but none of them had any reference to illnesses. Although 21 samples were later taken in an area mapped by the water company, no water quality issues were identified through on-site and laboratory testing and an assessment of the taste and odour descriptions reported by customers showed great variation. Therefore, the initial investigation was deemed inconclusive.

However, following discussions with another water company, which was experiencing a similar issue, it was determined that the unusual tastes and odours in the drinking water was associated with the presence of two compounds in the local storage reservoirs and river, where raw water was abstracted:

- 2-ethyl-5,5-dimethyl-1,3-dioxane (2-EDD)
- 2-ethyl-4-methyl-1,3-dioxolane (2-EMD)

2-EDD and 2-EMD are by-products of resin manufacture, while 2-EMD could also possibly be used in food products, for example wine. After further investigation, it was concluded that these compounds had entered the local river via a discrete commercial process stream, at the water company's sewage treatment works. Discharge from this process stream was ceased.

During the earlier stages of the reported incident, when the cause of the unusual tastes and odours in drinking water was still unknown, public health discussions were undertaken with CRCE, though at this stage, restriction of water use was not considered appropriate. Expert assessment of the detected low levels of 2-EDD and 2-EMD considered that there was little appreciable risk to human health but their presence in drinking water could result in taste and odour issues.

It was noted that the taste and odour descriptions of these compounds were likely to be very varied, for example fruity, musty, solvent, sweet, and so on. Following assessment of public health advice, the provision of alternative water supplies was not considered necessary.

During the incident, a number of symptoms were reported by customers from the affected area, such as headaches and gastrointestinal and skin complaints. However, it was deemed unlikely that consumption of drinking water contaminated with these compounds at low levels (see Table 5.3) would have resulted in such symptoms; it was more likely that the aesthetic issues encountered by customers resulted in a perception that they were responsible for symptoms experienced.

Table 5.3 Maximum levels observed for 2-EDD and 2-EMD during the incident

Contaminant	Maximum levels (µg/l)
2-EDD	0.026
2-EMD	0.186

Throughout the incident, the water company maintained frequent communication with CRCE and the regulators. This ensured continuing engagement with stakeholders and provision of consistent information to customers. Information was placed on the water company's website to inform customers of the incident. In addition, a number of press statements were issued by the water company, as well as a letter dispatched to all customers who had contacted the water company regarding the incident.

Summary

Experience in responding to chemical contamination in drinking water incidents has shown that, in order to provide effective support to the public and consumers, effective communication between public health organisations, water companies, the regulators, and other related bodies are essential elements for a successful response. In order to carry out effective risk assessments for water-related incidents, environmental public health professionals need to understand the sources and common water treatment techniques, the toxicology of chemicals likely to be present in water, and the regulatory framework, as illustrated in this chapter.

It is of great importance for the water industry to consider planning, preparation, and performance when assessing the impact of incidents affecting drinking water quality (Jackson, 2004). Planning must be thorough and capable of tackling the most unthinkable scenarios. Preparation must ensure that the provision of analytical facilities is adequate, with appropriate expertise to interpret the results of such analyses. In addition, good availability of safe alternative drinking water supplies and effective communication are essential to maintain public confidence during unexpected emergency situations.

Acknowledgement

We gratefully acknowledge the contribution of David Mason in the chemical pollutants section.

References

Agency for Toxic Substances and Disease Registry (ATSDR) (2002). *Toxicological Profile for Aldrin/dieldrin*. ATSDR, Atlanta. Available at: http://www.atsdr.cdc.gov/ToxProfiles/tp1.pdf [Accessed 28 February 2013].

Binnie, C. and Kimber, M. (2009). *Basic Water Treatment*. 4th ed. Thomas Telford Publishing, London.

Bouchard, M., Sauvé, S., Barbeau, B. et al. (2010). Intellectual impairment in school-age children exposed to manganese from drinking water. *Environmental Health Perspectives*, **119**:1, 138. Available at: http://www.ncbi.nlm.nih.gov/pmc/articles/PMC3018493/pdf/ehp-119-138.pdf [Accessed 28 February 2013].

Panel on Contaminants in the Food Chain (CONTAM) (2010). Scientific opinion on lead in food. *European Food Safety Authority Journal*, 8:4, 1570. Available at: http://www.efsa.europa.eu/en/search/doc/1570.pdf [Accessed 28 February 2013].

Committee on carcinogenicity of chemicals in food consumer products and the environment (COC) (2008). *Second Statement on Chlorinated Drinking Water and Cancer COC/08/S1*. Available at: http://www.iacoc.org.uk/statements/documents/SecondstatementonCBPsandcancerCOC08.S1.pdf [Accessed 28 February 2013].

Committee on toxicity of chemicals in food consumer products and the environment (COT) (2008). COT statement on a SAHSU Study on chlorination disinfection by-products and risk of congenital anomalies in England and Wales. Available at: http://cot.food.gov.uk/pdfs/cotstatementdbp200802.pdf [Accessed 28 February 2013].

Crittenden, J., Trussell, R., Hand, D. et al. (2012). *Water Treatment Principles and Design*. 3rd ed. John Wiley & Sons, Chichester.

Drinking Water Inspectorate (DWI) (2009). *Drinking Water Safety, Guidance to Health and Water Professionals*. DWI, London. Available at: http://dwi.defra.gov.uk/stakeholders/information-letters/2009/09_2009Annex.pdf [Accessed 28 February 2013].

Drinking Water Inspectorate (DWI) (2010). United Kingdom Drinking Water Regulators and the Environment Agency. Available at: http://dwi.defra.gov.uk/about/working-with-others/uk-ireland-mou.pdf [Accessed 7 June 2013].

Environment Agency (EA) (2012a). *Water*. EA, London. Available at: http://www.environment-agency.gov.uk/research/policy/40125.aspx [Accessed 28 February 2013].

Environment Agency (EA) (2012b). *Introduction to the Water Framework Directive*. EA, London. Available at: http://www.environment-agency.gov.uk/research/planning/33362.aspx [Accessed 28 February 2013].

European Food Safety Authority (2010). Conclusion on pesticide peer review—conclusion on the peer review of the pesticide risk assessment of the active substance carbetamide. *European Food Safety Authority Journal*, 8:12. Available at: http://www.efsa.europa.eu/en/search/doc/1913.pdf [Accessed 28 February 2013].

Food Standards Agency (FSA) (2003). *Safe Upper Levels for Vitamins and Minerals*. FSA, London. Available at: http://cot.food.gov.uk/pdfs/vitmin2003.pdf#page=186 [Accessed 28 February 2013].

Health Protection Agency (HPA) (2008). *Chemical Information Note: Metaldehyde*. HPA, Chilton.

HPA (2009). *Chemical Information Note: Clopyralid*. HPA, Chilton.

HPA (2011). *HPA Compendium of Chemical Hazards: Arsenic*. HPA, Chilton. Available at: http://www.hpa.org.uk/webc/HPAwebFile/HPAweb_C/1202487025752 [Accessed 28 February 2013].

HPA (2012a). *Private Water Supplies—Advice on the health impact associated with exceedances of the drinking-water quality standards*. HPA, Chilton.

HPA (2012b). *Lead—Toxicological review*. HPA, Chilton. Available at: http://www.hpa.org.uk/webc/HPAwebFile/HPAweb_C/1194947332124 [Accessed 28 February 2013].

International Agency for Research on Cancer (IARC) (2006). *IARC Monographs Volume 87: Inorganic and organic lead compounds*. IARC, Lyon. Available at: http://monographs.iarc.fr/ENG/Monographs/vol87/mono87-10.pdf [Accessed 28 February 2013].

IARC (2010). *Ingested Nitrate and Nitrite, and Cyanobacterial Peptide Toxins*. IARC, Lyon. Available at: http://monographs.iarc.fr/ENG/Monographs/vol94/mono94.pdf [Accessed 28 February 2013].

IPCS (1981a). *Environmental Health Criteria Monographs—Arsenic*. WHO, Geneva. Available at: http://www.inchem.org/documents/ehc/ehc/ehc018.htm#SubSectionNumber:3.1.3 [Accessed 28 February 2013].

IPCS (1981b). *Environmental Health Criteria Monographs—Manganese*. WHO, Geneva. Available at: http://www.inchem.org/documents/ehc/ehc/ehc017.htm#SectionNumber:10.1 [Accessed 28 February 2013].

IPCS (1986). *Environmental Health Criteria Monographs—Selenium*. WHO, Geneva. Available at: http://www.inchem.org/documents/ehc/ehc/ehc58.htm#SectionNumber:4.2 [Accessed 28 February 2013].

IPCS (1997). *Environmental Health Criteria Monographs—Aluminium*. WHO, Geneva. Available at: http://www.inchem.org/documents/ehc/ehc/ehc194.htm [Accessed 2 September 2013].

IPCS (1998a). *Environmental Health Criteria Monographs—Boron*. WHO, Geneva. Available at: http://www.inchem.org/documents/ehc/ehc/ehc204.htm#SectionNumber:3.1 [Accessed 28 February 2013].

IPCS (1998b). *Environmental Health Criteria Monographs—Copper*. WHO, Geneva. Available at: http://www.inchem.org/documents/ehc/ehc/ehc200.htm#SubSectionNumber:5.2.3 [Accessed 28 February 2013].

Jackson, C. (2004). Problems, perceptions and perfection—the role of the drinking water inspectorate in water quality incidents and emergencies. In: Thompson, K. C. and Gray, J. (Eds) *Water Contamination Emergencies: Can we cope?* pp 38–43. Royal Society of Chemistry, Cambridge.

Joint FAO/WHO Expert Committee on Food Additives (JECFA) (1983). *Monograph 571: Iron*. JECFA, Geneva. Available at: http://www.inchem.org/documents/jecfa/jecmono/v18je18.htm [Accessed 28 February 2013].

JECFA (2002). *WHO Food Additives Series: 50. Nitrate*. JECFA, Geneva. Available at: http://www.inchem.org/documents/jecfa/jecmono/v50je06.htm [Accessed 28 February 2013].

JECFA (2010). *Seventy-third Meeting, Geneva, 8–17 June 2012: Summary and conclusions*. JECFA, Geneva. Available at: http://www.who.int/foodsafety/publications/chem/summary73.pdf [Accessed 28 February 2013].

Krasner, S. (2009). The formation and control of emerging disinfection by-products of health concern. *Philosophical Transactions of the Royal Society A*, **367**, 4077–4095.

Manassaram, D., Backer, L., Messing, R. et al. (2010). Nitrates in drinking water and methemoglobin levels in pregnancy: A longitudinal study. *Environmental Health* **9**, 60. Available at: http://www.ncbi.nlm.nih.gov/pmc/articles/PMC2967503/ [Accessed 28 February 2013].

National Health Service (NHS) (2012). *What is NHS Direct?* NHS, London. Available at: http://www.nhsdirect.nhs.uk/About/WhatIsNHSDirect [Accessed 28 February 2013].

Private Water Supplies Regulations (2009). SI 2009/3101. HMSO, London.

Private Water Supplies (Wales) Regulations (2010). SI 2010/66. HMSO, London.

Scottish Executive (2006). *Private Water Supplies: Technical menu*. WHO, Edinburgh. Available at: http://www.privatewatersupplies.gov.uk/private_water/files/Full%20Doc.pdf [Accessed 28 February 2013].

Water Act (2003). (c.37). HMSO, London.

Water Industry Act (1991). (c.56). HMSO, London.

Water Supply (Water Quality) Regulations (2000). SI 2000/3184. HMSO, London.

World Health Organization (WHO) (2003a). *Aluminium in Drinking-water*. WHO, Geneva. Available at: http://www.who.int/water_sanitation_health/dwq/chemicals/en/aluminium.pdf [Accessed 28 February 2013].

WHO (2003b). *Iron in Drinking-water*. WHO, Geneva. Available at: http://www.who.int/water_sanitation_health/dwq/chemicals/iron.pdf [Accessed 28 February 2013].

WHO (2003c). *Aldrin and Dieldrin in Drinking-water*. WHO, Geneva. Available at: http://www.who.int/water_sanitation_health/dwq/chemicals/adrindieldrin.pdf [Accessed 28 February 2013].

WHO (2004a). *Copper in Drinking-water*. WHO, Geneva. Available at: http://www.who.int/water_sanitation_health/dwq/chemicals/copper.pdf [Accessed 28 February 2013].

WHO (2004b). *Vitamin and Mineral Requirements in Human Nutrition*. 2nd ed. WHO, Hong Kong. Available at: http://whqlibdoc.who.int/publications/2004/9241546123.pdf [Accessed 28 February 2013].

WHO (2009). *Boron in Drinking-water*. WHO, Geneva. Available at: http://whqlibdoc.who.int/hq/2009/WHO_HSE_WSH_09.01_2_eng.pdf [Accessed 28 February 2013].

WHO (2010). *Aluminium in Drinking-water*. WHO, Geneva. Available at: http://www.who.int/water_sanitation_health/dwq/chemicals/aluminium.doc [Accessed 28 February 2013].

WHO (2011a). *Guidelines for Drinking-water Quality*. 4th ed. WHO, Geneva. Available at: http://whqlibdoc.who.int/publications/2011/9789241548151_eng.pdf [Accessed 28 February 2013].

WHO (2011b). *Arsenic in Drinking-water*. WHO, Geneva. Available at: http://www.who.int/water_sanitation_health/dwq/chemicals/arsenic.pdf [Accessed 28 February 2013].

WHO (2011c). *Lead in Drinking-water*. WHO, Geneva. Available at: http://www.who.int/water_sanitation_health/dwq/chemicals/lead.pdf [Accessed 28 February 2013].

WHO (2011d). *Manganese in Drinking-water*. WHO, Geneva. Available at: http://www.who.int/water_sanitation_health/dwq/chemicals/manganese.pdf [Accessed 28 February 2013].

Chapter 6

Contaminated land and public health

Yolande Macklin, Kerry Foxall, Paul Harold, Louise Uffindell, Sian Morrow, and George Kowalczyk

Learning objectives

By the end of this chapter the reader will be able to:
- understand the current regulatory regime covering the assessment of potentially contaminated land in the UK
- understand the main soil contaminants and the main routes of exposure for the public
- understand the basic steps in land contamination risk assessment
- through case studies understand how to investigate, assess, and remediate land affected by contamination
- understand good practice in communicating risks to the public.

Introduction

Most of the land contamination in the developed world is the result of past and current industrial activity. Some naturally occurring substances may also represent a risk to health, for example, concentration of contaminants in soils due to the geology of some areas of the UK. However, the key question for public health professionals is whether the level of pollution is sufficient to present a risk to health. For example, exposure to soils rich in heavy metals such as cadmium and lead could have measurable and often severe effects on local populations.

Risk assessment of land affected by contamination can be very complex. Individual sites often have a long history of use, which may have left a mixture of contaminants in a variety of soil and ground types. Such contaminated sites may present a risk to people who currently use the site; however, any risk assessment undertaken may need to consider their likely future use/users. Furthermore, actual or perceived contamination may cause property blight leading to long-term dereliction.

This chapter will help the reader to understand the current legislative framework. Through the use of case studies, it also illustrates the key approaches to assessing and developing potentially contaminated land in the UK.

Sources and key pollutants

Industry has resulted in the deposition of many hazardous substances in the ground, including heavy metals, organic compounds, oils and tars, and soluble salts. Many soils have chemical contaminants present at low levels (caused by naturally complex geology and diffuse anthropogenic pollution) but the risks are generally low.

Many researchers have suggested a number of contaminants or groups of contaminants that may be key indicators of land contamination (see Table 6.1). It must be emphasised that any investigation must not rely solely on these key contaminants, as different historic land uses may result in different mixtures of pollutants. Table 6.2 gives examples of substances commonly associated with five major industrial processes. Other industry profiles are publicly available and provide developers, local authorities, and others with information on the processes, materials, and wastes associated with individual industries.

As is clearly shown in Tables 6.1 and 6.2, soil can be a source of exposure to heavy metals and organic pollutants such as polycyclic aromatic hydrocarbons (PAHs). The presence of such contaminants can pose risks to human health through direct ingestion or contact with contaminated soil, the food chain (soil-plant-human or soil-plant-animal-human), or groundwater pollution.

The risks presented by any given level of contaminant are usually assessed for each site, with consideration given to nearby sensitive receptors. Site-specific factors may include the current and proposed land usage, proximity to ground or surface water, or receptors in adjacent dwellings or habitats.

Many contaminants are typically due to a combination of natural and diffuse anthropogenic pollution, for example from activities associated with mining and associated processes. Therefore, estimating the contaminants' background concentrations is important when assessing risk. The British Geological Survey (BGS) (Johnson et al., 2012) was commissioned by the Department for Environment, Food and Rural Affairs (Defra) to provide guidance as to what Normal Background Concentrations (NBC) could be expected for soils in England. The project considered eight key contaminants: arsenic, benzo(a)pyrene, cadmium, chromium, copper, lead, mercury, and nickel.

This project highlighted that there was a large variability in contaminant concentrations. Much of this variability can be attributed to the underlying parent material on which a soil has formed. The project clearly showed that certain contaminants are ubiquitous in the urban environment, for example lead, which is at much higher levels in urban settings partly due to historic emissions of leaded fuels from vehicles.

As part of the project, national soil contaminant maps were published together with contaminant-specific technical guidance sheets. This information provides a best effort to

Table 6.1 Key soil contaminants in the UK

Inorganic contaminants	Organic contaminants
Metals	Acetone
Barium	Oil/fuel hydrocarbons
Beryllium	**Aromatic hydrocarbons**
Cadmium	Benzene
Chromium	Chlorophenols
Copper	Ethylbenzene
Lead	Phenol
Mercury	Toluene
Nickel	o-Xylene
Vanadium	Polycyclic aromatic hydrocarbons
Zinc	**Chlorinated aliphatic hydrocarbons**
Semi-metals and non-metals	Chloroform
Arsenic	Carbon tetrachloride
Boron	Vinyl chloride
Selenium	1,2-Dichloroethane
Sulphur	1,1,1-Trichloroethane
Inorganic chemicals	Trichloroethene
Cyanide (complex)	Tetrachloroethene
Cyanide (free)	Hexachlorobuta-1,3-diene
Nitrate	Hexachlorocyclohexanes
Sulfate	Dieldrin
Sulfide	**Chlorinated aromatic hydrocarbons**
Other	Chlorobenzenes
Asbestos	Chlorotoluenes
pH (acidity/alkalinity)	Pentachlorophenol
	Polychlorinated biphenyls
	Dioxins and furans
	Organometallics
	Organolead compounds
	Organotin compounds

Adapted from Kibble, A. and Russell, D., Contaminated land and health, pp. 565–573, in: Ayres, J. G. et al., (Eds) *Environmental Medicine*. CRC Press, Copyright © 2010 with permission from Taylor & Francis Group, LLC. All Rights Reserved.

Table 6.2 Examples of contaminants associated with specific industries

Industry/process	Potentially contaminating substances
Chemical works	Solvents, phenols, benzoic acid, cadmium, mercury, hexavalent chromium, vanadium
Oil refineries	Fuel oils, lubricants, bitumen, alcohols, organic acids, PCBs, cyanides, sulphur, vanadium
Lead works	Lead, arsenic, cadmium, sulfides, sulfates, chlorides, sulphuric acid, sodium hydroxide
Timber treatment works	Organochlorines, phenolics, organotin compounds, metal carboxylates, pyrethroids, creosote, copper, arsenic, kerosene
Textile and dye works	Aluminium, cadmium, mercury, bromides, fluorides, ammonium salts, trichloroethane, polyvinyl chloride

Source: Data from Department of the Environment Industry Profiles © Crown Copyright 1995, licensed under the Open Government Licence v1.0, available from http://www.environment-agency.gov.uk/research/planning/33708.aspx.

define the upper limit of NBC in soil as described by the contaminated land statutory guidance. These documents are not intended to be used for urban planning or as a bespoke risk assessment tool but can help to provide information on the quality of land.

Legislation and legal framework

The current government policy on land contamination is built on a dual principle of preventing new areas of land being affected by contamination (for example accidental chemical spills or through deposition of air pollutants), whilst taking into account a risk-based approach for tackling historical contamination. The former is discussed in earlier chapters; the discussion in this chapter focusses on the legislation concerning tackling historical contamination.

There are many different terms used to describe land affected by contamination. Table 6.3 gives an indication of some of the common terminology that may be encountered and its meaning.

Most of the contamination to land occurred prior to the introduction of regulations to control waste disposal and polluting practices (for example Control of Pollution Act 1974). In the UK, there are two key pieces of legislation requiring the risk assessment of land contamination:

- Part 2A Environmental Protection Act 1990 (enacted in 1995)
- Town and Country Planning Act 1990.

These two acts are discussed in detail later in this chapter but it is important to note that, whilst they may be different, the underlying approach to identifying and dealing with risk and the broad policy objective of safeguarding human health and the environment are similar. The sections that follow concentrate on the aspects relating to human health.

Table 6.3 Common terminology used to describe land affected by contamination

Brownfield land	A term generally used to describe post-industrial land that may have been subjected to potentially contaminating land uses. This term is often used in the planning context.
Greenfield land	A term reserved for land not previously developed. Greenfields are not necessarily free from contamination. There are known instances where waste disposal practices (for example, spreading of wastes to nearby land), agricultural practices, or the spread of chemicals from natural processes have resulted in contamination of greenfield sites.
Contaminated land	Land that meets the definition set down in Part 2A of the Environmental Protection Act 1990 (often simply referred to as Part IIA or Part 2A). Therefore, the term 'contaminated' does not automatically apply to land simply because it is known to contain contaminants.

Text extracts reproduced from Health Protection Agency, *An Introduction to Land Contamination for Public Health Professionals*, p. 2, Copyright © 2009, with permission from Public Health England, available from: http://www.hpa.org.uk/webc/HPAwebFile/HPAweb_C/1242198452810.

The legislation requires a risk assessment based on the contaminant (source)-pathway-receptor approach:

- **Contaminant**: a substance that is in, on, or under the land that has the potential to cause harm to human health or the environment, or to cause pollution of controlled waters.
- **Pathway**: a route or means by which a receptor could be exposed to a contaminant.
- **Receptor**: includes any person or ecosystem potentially impacted by a contaminant.

All three must be present for a risk to occur and this is usually called a contaminant or pollutant linkage.

It may not always be necessary for legislative mechanisms to be used to drive the clean-up (remediation) of contaminated sites. There have been many instances where companies have undertaken voluntary remediation of sites due to public concern or as part of an assessment of liabilities within a company's land holdings.

Town and Country Planning Act 2010

The EA have estimated that, in England, 87 per cent of land affected by contamination is dealt with through planning, 4 per cent through voluntary mechanism, and 9 per cent through Part 2A (Environment Agency, 2009a). The role of the planning system is to control future development and land uses; it is managed by the Local Planning Authority (which sits within the local authority). The contaminated land identified through this regulatory regime is risk assessed, and if necessary remediated, before it is redeveloped. The planning process is enforced by imposing conditions on the planning permission issued by the Local Planning Authority.

A piece of land in its current state may not pose a risk to human health or the environment but redevelopment may introduce new receptors or pathways that may result in new contaminant linkages. Case Study 6.1 gives an example of this.

Case Study 6.1: Example of redevelopment of land introducing pathways to human health

Site A was a former waste tip and industrial site covering approximately 8 ha. The site was previously used for a mixture of light industry and public open space. Large areas of the site were contaminated with heavy metals resulting from use as an unregulated waste tip prior to building the current light industrial units. Users of the site had limited contact with the soil due to vegetative and hardcover; therefore they were not exposed to the underlying soils.

The land was being risk assessed before being redeveloped for housing. The presence of houses on the site meant that people could be exposed to much more of the soil (for example by exposing bare soil for gardening and eating home-grown vegetables). Therefore, planning conditions were placed on the developer, requiring site remediation so that pollution did not present a significant risk of harm to future occupants.

The developer is responsible for ensuring that a development is safe and that the land is suitable for the use intended. After remediation has been carried out, developers must prove to the Local Planning Authority that it has been successful by, for example, submitting a verification report demonstrating that the risk associated with land contamination has been reduced to meet the remediation objectives.

It is important to note that any site remediated under the Town and Country Planning Act 1990 should not need to be determined as contaminated land under Part 2A Environmental Protection Act 1990 (Communities and Local Government, 2012).

The planning rules are overseen by the Department for Communities and Local Government. The planning policy was devolved in 1999; Scotland and Wales operate systems similar to England's.

Part 2A Environmental Protection Act

Part 2A came into force on 1 April 2000 in England and on 15 September 2001 in Wales, with the production of the first version of the Statutory Guidance. Policy was devolved in 1999; Scotland and Wales operate systems similar to England's. The system is not yet in force in Northern Ireland.

Part 2A focusses on the identification and remediation of land that in its current use poses an unacceptable risk to people or the environment. It is designed to deal with the most seriously contaminated sites that would not be remediated by any other mechanism (i.e. where nothing would be done without regulatory intervention). The act places key responsibilities on the local authorities for the identification, assessment, and remediation of contaminated land (see the section on Roles and responsibilities).

Part 2A is a complex piece of legislation that has undergone considerable changes over the last 10 years. Defra recently undertook a review of the contaminated land regime in

> **Box 6.1 Legal definition of contaminated land for England as laid down in Part 2A of the Environmental Protection Act 1990**
>
> Section 78A(2): 'Contaminated land' is any land which appears to the local authority in whose area it is situated to be in such a condition, by reason of substances in, on or under the land, that—
>
> a. significant harm is being caused or there is a significant possibility of such harm being caused; or
>
> b. pollution of controlled waters is being, or is likely to be, caused.
>
> Reproduced from Environmental Protection Act 1990, licensed under the Open Government Licence v1.0.

England, to assess whether any improvements could be made to the regime based on the experiences of the last 10 years of delivery. The review concluded that the primary legislation was fit for purpose but that there were flaws in the accompanying Statutory Guidance (SG) that created considerable regulatory uncertainty. In April 2012, Defra published a simpler and shorter version of the Statutory Guidance to allow regulators to make more rapid decisions about whether or not land is contaminated under Part 2A (Defra, 2012) (see Box 6.1).

The risk assessment process is detailed later in this chapter. For the land to be declared 'contaminated land', there must be a 'significant contaminant linkage'; i.e. the level of risk must result in 'significant harm' or a 'significant possibility of significant harm' (SPOSH). The Part 2A Contaminated Land SG provides definitions of what is considered significant harm or SPOSH (Defra, 2012).

The revised version of the SG introduced a more targeted approach, with a new category system ranging from Category 4 (no risk or the level of risk posed is acceptably low) to Category 1 (where the level of risk is clearly unacceptable and 'significant harm' is occurring) (see Figure 6.1 and Box 6.2). The boundary between Categories 2 and 3 represents the point beyond which the land can be defined as contaminated. It is often a complicated decision, and the SG details a number of variables the local authorities should consider before making their decision. This includes: the likelihood of harm to the identified receptor; the impact, i.e. the nature and seriousness of the harm; and (where relevant) the extent of the harm in terms of how many people may be affected. Other factors that may need to be taken into account are: socio-economic factors; the direct and indirect health benefits; impacts of regulatory intervention; and whether the benefits would outweigh the financial and economic costs.

The terms 'contaminant', 'pollutant', and 'substance' as used in the SG and non-statutory guidance have the same meaning, i.e. a substance relevant to the Part 2A regime.

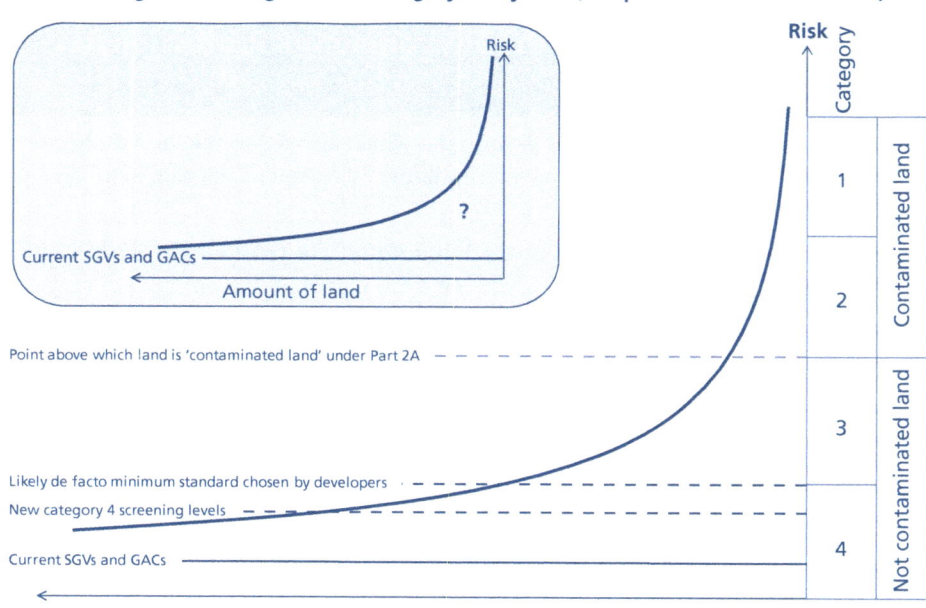

Fig. 6.1 Diagram showing the new Category 1–4 system.

Reproduced from *Simplification of the Contaminated Land Regime: Impact Assessment*, Defra (Department for Environment, Food and Rural Affairs) and Cranfield University © Crown Copyright 2011, licensed under the Open Government Licence v1.0, available from http://archive.defra.gov.uk/environment/quality/land/contaminated/documents/contaminated-land-ia.pdf.

Box 6.2 Definition of significant harm as detailed in Section 4.1 of the Statutory Guidance (Defra, 2012)

Always constitutes significant harm
  Death
  Life-threatening diseases (cancer)
  Other diseases likely to have serious impacts on health; serious injury; birth defects; and impairment of reproductive functions

May constitute significant harm*
  Physical injury
  Gastrointestinal disturbances
  Respiratory tract effects
  Cardiovascular effects
  Central nervous system effects
  Skin ailments

> **Box 6.2 Definition of significant harm as detailed in Section 4.1 of the Statutory Guidance (Defra, 2012)** *(continued)*
>
> Effects on organs such as the liver or kidney
>
> Or a wide range of other health impacts
>
> *Local authority can make the decision as to whether it may or may not be significant harm (alone or in combination). The statutory guidance states that when deciding whether or not a particular form of harm is significant harm, the local authority should consider the seriousness of the harm in question, including the impact on health and quality of life of any person suffering the harm, and the scale of the harm.
>
> Source: Data from Environmental Protection Act 1990: Part 2A Contaminated Land Statutory Guidance, Defra (Department for Environment, Food and Rural Affairs) © Crown Copyright 2012, licensed under the Open Government Licence v1.0, available from https://www.gov.uk/government/publications/contaminated-land-statutory-guidance.

The SG also details that reasonable use of the land, which does not require planning permission, should be considered. For example, if a residential house currently has a garden but it is completely paved, there is currently no pathway to the soil. However, under Part 2A, the local authority must take into account that the current or future resident may wish to remove the paving slabs, exposing the soil

The idea is that, where 'contaminated land' sites are identified, the local authority must ensure reasonable remediation is undertaken and decide who will pay. The underlying principle is that the polluter should pay; however, the polluter is not always traceable. In this case, the current owner may be required to pay. In cases where no one else can be found, the local authority may have to meet the remediation costs.

Roles and responsibilities

Local authorities

As mentioned earlier in this chapter, local authorities are the principal regulators for contaminated land and have sole responsibility for the identification of contaminated land under Part 2A, within their area. Only local authorities can formally determine land as 'contaminated land'; they have a duty to inspect their local area from time to time and identify any areas that may fit the legal definition of contaminated land. Local authorities must provide a publicly available register of regulatory actions taken in regard to contaminated land sites.

However, some sites can be designated by the local authority as 'special sites' (see Box 6.3). The regulatory responsibility for these sites will pass to the Environment Agency (EA) in England if they agree that the site falls under the conditions for 'special sites'. (In Wales and Scotland this responsibility lies with Natural Resources Wales and the Scottish Environmental Protection Agency, respectively.) The local authority is also responsible for consulting with the EA on the pollution of controlled waters.

In addition to their responsibilities under the Part 2A legislation, Local Planning Authorities may place planning conditions that should ensure that any contamination of a

> **Box 6.3 Definition of special sites**
>
> Special sites are particular sites that meet a specific set of conditions described within the Part 2A regulations. They include:
>
> - Some water pollution cases: includes areas of contaminated land affecting drinking water supply or (potentially) controlled waters within a primary aquifer.
> - Industrial cases: includes specific circumstances such as acid tar lagoons, sites where explosives were manufactured, or a site for an authorized process under the Environmental Permitting (England and Wales) Regulations and its predecessor regimes.
> - Defence cases: including most land currently owned by the Ministry of Defence and by visiting forces.
> - Radioactivity cases: where land is contaminated land by virtue of radioactivity, which can include nuclear sites.
>
> Source: Data from Environmental Protection Act 1990: Part 2A Contaminated Land Statutory Guidance, Defra (Department for Environment, Food and Rural Affairs) © Crown Copyright 2012, licensed under the Open Government Licence v1.0, available from https://www.gov.uk/government/publications/contaminated-land-statutory-guidance.

site is properly remediated. These conditions will not be discharged until the authority is satisfied that their requirements have been met by the developer.

Environment Agency (EA)

The EA are responsible for the regulation of 'special sites' and for the maintenance of a register of regulatory action on such sites (see Box 6.3). The EA has a role in providing site-specific advice to local authorities regarding pollution of controlled waters by contaminated land. The EA also manages funding for the Contaminated Land Capital Projects Programme, on behalf of Defra, to help local authorities in England cover the cost of implementing contaminated land legislation.

The EA will also from time to time publish research or technical guidance that can be referred to. These publications cover a wider range of topics relevant to land contamination. The most notable publication is probably the *Model Procedures for the Management of Land Contamination* (CLR11) (Defra and Environment Agency, 2004), which sets out a general framework for good practice in land contamination management and the steps that should be followed. In addition, the EA have published guidance on assessing risks to human health on sites affected by contamination.

Department for the Environment, Food and Rural Affairs (Defra)

The role of Defra is to prepare land contamination policy. In England, Defra are responsible for the provision of statutory guidance and funding for the Contaminated Land Capital

Projects Programme. The devolved administrations are responsible for statutory guidance and funding for contaminated land in their areas.

Defra also fund a number of studies to assist with the development of guidance for the contaminated land industry. Most recently, this has included a research project to provide assessment criteria to define what is definitely not considered to be contaminated land under Part 2A (Category 4 screening levels). Defra also funded the British Geological Survey (BGS) to undertake research on the typical background concentrations of selected contaminants in soils in England.

Other government agencies

Other government bodies that may be involved with the investigation of land contamination include the Food Standards Agency (FSA) and Animal Health and Veterinary Laboratories Agency (AHVLA). The FSA can provide technical and public health advice where the consumption of produce on land affected by contamination is involved, for example allotments or agricultural land use. The AHVLA can provide technical advice on potential risks to livestock (which are a receptor under Part 2A) from land contamination, for example agricultural land or a horse paddock.

Site developers/Site owners

Under the planning regime, it is the responsibility of the developer or site owner to ensure that the site is fit for the purpose for which planning permission is being sought. This includes ensuring any remedial actions required as part of the planning consent are carried out.

As Part 2A operates a 'polluter pays' policy, the current or previous site owners may be liable for the remediation if the local authority deems the land to be 'contaminated land' in the legal sense of the term.

Public health professionals

Public health professionals, such as those in Public Health England, Public Health Wales, or Directors of Public Health within Local Authorities, can provide additional expertise in carrying out human health risk assessments and assisting with the risk communication activities for concerned communities and members of the public. Where land contamination is suspected to be causing health effects amongst a particular community, public health professionals can assist in collating and interpreting data on the health of the population under investigation.

Risk assessment

The UK operates a risk-based approach to assessing land contamination and risk assessments are required as part of the assessment process for establishing whether land is 'contaminated land'. Defra and the EA have published guidance to assist in the steps required in a risk assessment. These steps are laid out the CLR11 *Model Procedures for the Management of Land Contamination* (Defra, 2004). Essentially, this document recommends a tiered approach to risk assessment:

- Tier 1: Preliminary risk assessment (PRA)
- Tier 2: Generic quantitative risk assessment (GQRA)
- Tier 3: Detailed quantitative risk assessment (DQRA)

Progression through all three tiers will not always take place; it depends on the findings of the earlier stages. At any point in the process it may not be necessary to conduct further investigations, or it may only be necessary to carry out further investigations on sections of the site or reduced numbers of contaminants. The decision making process is much the same for each tier, with aspects examined further or removed from the investigation after each stage or iteration.

Each of the three tiers is discussed in the following sections. The discussion only focusses on risks to human health at sites affected by contamination but there may be other receptors (for example groundwater) that need to be considered.

Tier 1: Preliminary risk assessment

The purpose of the preliminary risk assessment (PRA) is to develop an initial conceptual model for the site. The conceptual site model (CSM) is central to the whole risk assessment process and is vital for identifying whether there are any unacceptable risks to humans or the environment. The CSM represents the characteristics of the site in diagrammatic or written form, showing the possible relationships between contaminants, pathways, and receptors (contaminant linkages). An example of a conceptual model is shown in Figure 6.2.

The PRA is also commonly known as a 'desk-study', 'desk-top study', or 'Phase 1'. It largely involves collecting desk-based information on the site to make an initial assessment of the possible ground conditions and to review current and past history to create the initial CSM. Understanding the history of a site is key to understanding the potential for contaminants to be present on a site and their particular location if they are present.

The documents collected as part of the desk study include historical maps and aerial photographs. The EA can provide data on licensable activities (for example environmental permits) and local authorities hold information on historical landfill records and planning documentation. It is also possible to obtain records from commercial suppliers who will collate all the information sources.

The outcome of the PRA will be a report that discusses all the desk study information collected, presents an initial conceptual model, and provides any recommendations for further assessment at the site. The PRA will often also include a qualitative assessment that allows an initial ranking of the risk from the plausible 'contaminant linkages' as negligible, low, medium, or high risk. The overall ranking of risk is usually estimated from the potential severity of the linkage and the probability of it occurring (Defra and Cranfield University, 2011).

If any plausible 'contaminant linkages' are identified in the PRA, the assessment will progress to Tier 2 GQRA. The GQRA is informed by gathering information on the site

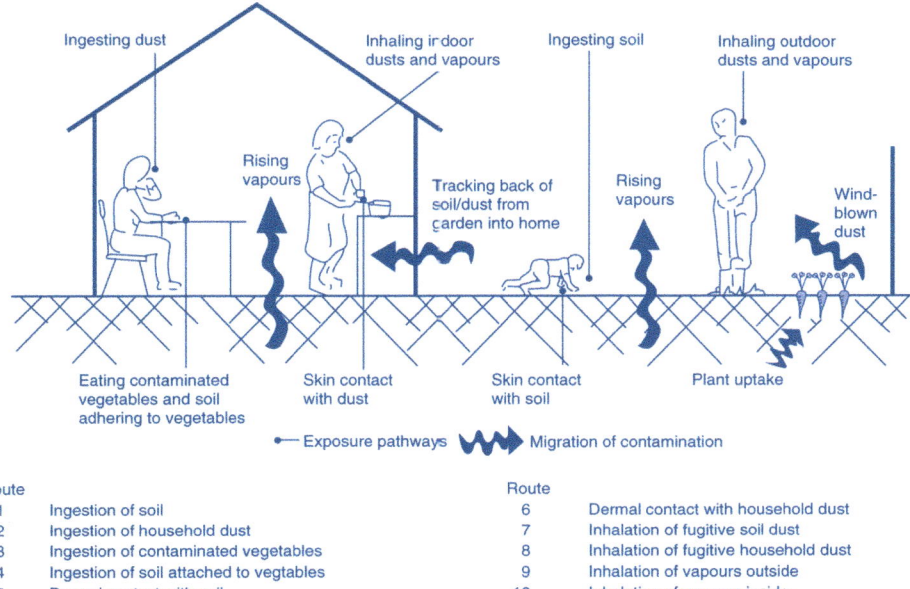

Fig. 6.2 Standard residential conceptual model (EA, 2009c).

Reproduced with permission from *Updated Technical Background to the CLEA model, Science Report SC050021/SR3*, Figure 2.1, p.14, Environment Agency, Copyright © 2009, available from http://www.environment-agency.gov.uk/static/documents/Research/CLEA_Report_-_final.pdf. Contains Environment Agency information © Environment Agency and database right.

through a site investigation. A site investigation will usually involve the collection of soil and possibly other media (for example groundwater) (depending on the pathways in the conceptual model) to inform the risk assessment. These samples are sent for detailed chemical analysis, which is usually targeted based on the chemicals anticipated to be present on the site.

Tier 2: Generic quantitative risk assessment (GQRA)

The GQRA is a process for determining whether contaminant linkages from the conceptual model can be screened out using generic assumptions about the behaviour of contaminants and receptors on site. The preliminary screening is through comparing site contaminant concentrations with Generic Assessment Criteria (GAC). GAC are criteria used in risk assessment that have been derived using generic assumptions about the characteristics of the source, pathway, and receptor. These generic assumptions relate to characteristics such as soil organic carbon content, exposure duration, and body weight and age of receptor.

The basic principle used to establish GAC is that they are set at the soil concentration where the Average Daily Exposure (ADE) from soil sources by a particular exposure route equals the Health Criteria Value (HCV). The ADE is calculated from the generic receptor and source assumptions described previously and the HCV is a toxicological value that is selected to be protective of chronic risks to health.

Primarily, when we assess land contamination we are interested in understanding the chronic (i.e. long-term) risk to health. This is because many of the contaminants will take many years to affect health. There are a few exceptions; where there are particularly high concentrations of contaminants it may be necessary to consider whether an immediate effect is occurring, or if a particular contaminant is present that can be toxic at low concentrations (such as cyanide). An example of this is presented in Case Study 6.2.

The EA issued best practice guidance to assist in the process of assessment of human health risks at potentially contaminated sites. The Soil Guideline Values (SGVs) are GACs for standard land uses (residential, commercial, and allotments) for a limited number of contaminants. A software tool called the Contaminated Land Exposure Assessment (CLEA) model has been published to allow users to derive GACs.

There are also two core documents published by the EA: the *Updated Technical Background to the CLEA model* (known as SR3; EA, 2009c) and *Human Health Toxicological Assessment of Contaminants in Soil* (known as SR2; EA, 2009b). SR3 provides the technical basis for the CLEA model. SR2 describes the framework for the collation and review of toxicological data and its subsequent use in the derivation of soil contaminant intakes (HCVs) that are considered to be protective of human health. These two documents in combination set out the technical approach that underpins the derivation of SGVs for use in the UK.

As the SGVs/GAC are based on generic assumptions, it is important that the risk assessor checks that they are applicable for the conceptual model at the site and will be sufficiently protective against the potential risks to health. Examples of when they might not be suitable are:

- additional pathways are present that are not considered in the SGV/GAC (see the section on Unusual exposure routes)
- the source characteristics of the contamination are different, for example contamination is at a shallower depth
- receptor exposure is greater, for example more prolonged contact with the soil than assumed in the SGV/GAC.

If GACs are appropriate for application to the identified potential contaminant linkages, it is possible at this stage to establish whether there are potentially unacceptable risks from the land contamination or to screen out sites. The assessor will refine the conceptual model and may either confirm or exclude potential pollutant linkages, or highlight new potential linkages identified during the assessment process. As with the PRA, the result will highlight what aspects must be investigated further to examine any remaining uncertainties. Following the GQRA, it may be possible to establish that the land is unlikely to represent a potential risk to health. However, if the GQRA suggests that the possibility of health risks remains or the GAC are not appropriate, then a DQRA or further site investigation may be necessary to establish if any risks to health exist. Case Study 6.2 provides an example of an acute risk assessment for a site affected by contamination.

Case Study 6.2: An example of an acute risk assessment for a site affected by contamination

Site B is an informal open space that is used regularly by dog walkers and pedestrians as a short cut. The site was an area that had historically been used as a tip for wastes from the nearby gas manufacturing plant. The waste product from the removal of hydrogen sulfide and hydrogen cyanide from manufactured gas was often referred to as 'blue billy' owing to its distinctive 'blue-green' colouration.

The site was investigated to determine if it met the definition of 'contaminated land' as set out in the Environmental Protection Act 1990. A site investigation was conducted that indicated that there were high concentrations of 'free cyanide' (also called easily liberated cyanide) within the blue deposits. During the investigation, it was noted that these blue deposits were present at the soil surface. This raised concerns due to the potentially acute risk to young children, as they may seek out the blue coloured materials, which were potentially much higher in free cyanide content.

There is widespread awareness that cyanide compounds are acutely toxic to humans and that lethal effects follow quickly after ingestion of relatively small amounts (i.e. a few grams). In the UK, there is no standard procedure for the human acute health risk assessment for cyanide contamination in soils. Therefore, an approach was devised by local public health professionals to examine what the risk would be from a child ingesting a one-off dose of this material. The assessment indicated that, if a child weighing 10 kg ingested 5 g of the cyanide material (with a concentration of 1545 mg kg^{-1}, the maximum concentration on site), this could result in a toxic dose when compared to toxicological data (i.e. Lowest Observed Adverse Effect Levels, LOAELs). The site was subsequently determined as 'contaminated land' and has now been remediated.

Tier 3: Detailed quantitative risk assessment

The DQRA is similar to the GQRA; however, it uses more detailed information (which may be collected during the site investigation) on the source and receptor characteristics to allow deviation from the generic assumption. Some of the common deviations from generic assumptions are adjustment of the exposure frequency (days per year exposed), incorporation of bioaccessibility-based estimates of bioavailability, and adjustment of soil organic matter content. The assessment criteria produced from the DQRA are usually called site specific assessment criteria (SSAC).

If there are exposure pathways present that are not within the CLEA model, for example inhalation of vapours from groundwater, it may be necessary to use a different risk assessment model to derive the SSACs. There are several tools that are commercially available, including Risk Based Corrective Action (RBCA) and Risk Integrated Software for Clean-ups (RISC). However, as these are US-derived risk assessment tools, they require significant modification to make them suitable for use in the UK context. Where site specific data is used, the assessor should provide full justification for the assumptions adopted.

The findings of the DQRA may be sufficient to estimate the potential risk to health, but on occasions further investigation and risk assessment are required. Where the risks have been adequately defined and a potential risk to health identified, the next step is usually to review the options for remediating the site ('options appraisal').

An example of how a site can progress through the tiers to DQRA is illustrated in Case Study 6.3.

Case Study 6.3: Example of a tiered risk assessment

Site C is a small housing estate located on the site of a former gas works. It was being assessed by the local authority as part of their duty under Part 2A, Environmental Protection Act 1990.

Tier 1: Preliminary risk assessment

A preliminary assessment of the site was undertaken by the local authority. This involved a desk study and a site walkover. They also undertook some limited sampling across the site. The information gathered included:

- Historic maps showing that a gas works was present from 1870–1969 and houses were built on the site in approximately 1973.
- Historic maps and plans of the site indicating that there were tar tanks and purifier beds present in the location where four of the houses on the estate are now located. The remaining houses were located on a former yard area.
- There was no evidence that the old structures had been removed from the site and no records of any remediation undertaken.
- Limited soil sampling from within the historical boundary showed elevated levels of heavy metals, volatile organic compounds (VOCs), in particular benzene, and polycyclic aromatic hydrocarbons (PAHs).

The preliminary risk assessment report concluded that there was a potentially significant contaminant linkage between the residential receptors living within the footprint of the site and contaminants that could be in the soil due to its former use. The conceptual model identified a number of exposure pathways, including ingestion of soil and inhalation of vapours. Recommendations were made to undertake further intrusive work and laboratory analysis in order to investigate the potential risks to those properties within the footprint.

Tier 2: Generic quantitative risk assessment

A consultant was contracted by the local authority to conduct an intrusive site investigation. This involved soil samples being taken from the front and rear of each of the properties. The consultant also installed boreholes on the site to allow samples of the groundwater to be taken. The samples were sent off to a specialist laboratory for analysis.

The consultant used SGVs and GACs derived using CLEA for residential land use with gardens to assess the concentrations of contaminants in the soil. In some soil samples a number of contaminants exceeded the SGVs/GACs, including arsenic, lead, benzene, and benzo(a)pyrene (BaP).

Statistical analysis was undertaken to calculate a 'representative concentration' of contaminants present at the site. The statistical analysis indicated 'hotspots' were present for BaP and benzene, but that the other exceedances were spatially isolated and would not correspond to an overall level of intake that would require further investigation. The 'hotspots' required further examination using site-specific criteria.

Tier 3: Detailed quantitative risk assessment

The conceptual model was refined following the GQRA. The main exposure pathways requiring further assessment were ingestion of soil for BaP and inhalation of vapours indoors for benzene. Site specific assessment criteria (SSAC) were developed for BaP and benzene using information on the soil conditions and receptor characteristics. Comparison of the hotspot concentrations of BaP to the SSAC indicated that it no longer exceeded the limits and therefore did not pose a risk to health. However, there was still an exceedance for benzene.

As the main exposure pathway for benzene was through inhalation of vapours inside the home, the local authority requested that the consultant undertake indoor air monitoring using adsorption tubes. The results of the indoor air monitoring indicated that the benzene concentration potentially could pose a risk to health. Therefore 'significant possibility of significant harm' (SPOSH) was established and the land on which two of the worst affected houses were built was determined to be contaminated land. The remaining houses were not considered to meet the conditions of SPOSH.

The exposure pathway was severed by the fitting of vapour-proof membranes in the houses' sub-floor void.

Toxicological aspects

Toxicological considerations form a critical part of the land contamination risk assessment process. When assessing the potential health risks of land contamination it is important to have an understanding of the toxicological properties (for example, carcinogenicity, genotoxicity, organ toxicity, reproductive toxicity, and teratogenicity) of the contaminants.

In the UK, toxicological data is used to derive health HCVs, which are soil intake values that are considered to be protective of human health. HCVs are guidelines on the level of long-term human exposure to individual chemicals in soil that are tolerable or pose a minimal risk. They are a key component in the derivation of SGVs and/or other generic or site-specific assessment criteria. HCVs are derived for oral and inhalation routes of exposure. There is rarely enough data to derive a HCV for dermal exposures; therefore the oral HCV is used to assess the risk from dermal exposure.

Evidence from occupational and environmental epidemiological studies and data on the mechanisms of absorption, transport, metabolism, and toxicity of chemicals within the human body are reviewed and considered in the derivation of HCVs. For some contaminants there are limited or no human data available; therefore the chemical risk assessment often relies on the use of experimental animal data. Toxicological evaluations by authoritative bodies can be used to inform the risk assessment of contaminants and in some cases it may be appropriate to use the HCVs developed by these groups (Environment Agency, 2009b).

When deriving HCVs it is important to distinguish between contaminants that display threshold and non-threshold effects.

Threshold toxicity

For contaminants that exhibit threshold effects a tolerable daily intake value (TDI) is used to derive the HCV. The TDI is defined as an estimate of the amount of chemical, expressed on a body weight basis (for example mg kg^{-1} bw day^{-1}), that can be ingested daily over a lifetime without appreciable health risk. The TDI concept was originally used in food safety but has been adapted to address exposure from other routes, such as inhalation and dermal contact. A TDI is derived by applying uncertainty factors to a point of departure (POD) identified from the toxicity data; this is typically data from animal studies. The uncertainty factors are applied to the POD to account for the uncertainties in extrapolating data from an animal study or test population to derive a HCV. The POD is usually a 'no observed adverse effect level' (NOAEL) or a benchmark dose (BMD) for the critical adverse effects. The BMD is derived by mathematically modelling the dose-response curve and estimating the BMD that gives a predetermined change in response (generally 5 or

10 per cent) when compared to background. The statistical 95 per cent lower confidence limit of the BMD, known as the BMDL, is usually used as the POD in the derivation of HCVs. An exceedance of the TDI is undesirable but does not necessarily mean that an adverse effect will occur. It is important to remember that the TDI itself is not a threshold for effect. The likelihood of adverse health effects occurring as a result of an exposure that exceeds the TDI requires expert judgement and should only be considered on a case-by-case basis. Factors that should be taken into account include the size and the duration of the exceedance, the steepness of the dose-response curve, and the effect that the TDI is based on (Environment Agency, 2009b).

Background exposure to the contaminant from other sources (i.e. food, drinking water, and air) is also accounted for when setting SGVs/GAC for threshold compounds. Mean daily intake (MDI) values are estimated for oral exposure (MDI_{oral}) and inhalation exposure (MDI_{inh}). The identified TDI and MDI are used to derive a tolerable daily soil intake (TDSI). The TDSI is equal to the TDI minus the MDI, except in cases where the MDI exceeds 50 per cent of the TDI, in which case the TDSI is arbitrarily set at 50 per cent of the TDI (Environment Agency, 2009b).

Non-threshold toxicity

For non-threshold contaminants, which carry some risk at any level of exposure, an index dose (ID) is derived as the HCV. An index dose is defined as an estimate of the amount of a chemical (expressed as a daily intake dose) that can be experienced over a lifetime with minimal health risk. The approach used to derive an ID for non-threshold carcinogens will depend upon the toxicological data available. Data from animal carcinogenicity bioassays can be used to derive a BMD. The application of a default value of 10,000 to the $BMDL_{10}$ is recommended to be a suitable margin. Where suitable human cancer data are available, quantitative dose-response modelling can be used to derive an ID (Environment Agency, 2009b).

The principle described applies to genotoxic carcinogens. However, other adverse effects may not exhibit a threshold of effect; for example, there is no evidence for a threshold for critical lead-induced effects including neurodevelopmental toxicity in children. For other non-threshold effects the approach adopted to derive a HCV will be dependent upon the chemical and the critical adverse effect (Environment Agency, 2009b).

Although the ID is a dose that corresponds to minimal risk, the ALARP (as low as reasonably practicable) principle applies to non-threshold contaminants, as they may pose a risk at any level of exposure. If an ID is exceeded, there will be an increased risk to health. The significance of the increased risk requires expert judgement and is often unquantifiable. When deriving a SGV/GAC for non-threshold contaminants, background exposure from other sources is not taken into consideration; this is consistent with current standard practice (Environment Agency, 2009a; b).

Further information on toxicological aspects of land contamination can be found in *Human Health Toxicological Assessment of Contaminants in Soil* (Environment Agency, 2009b).

Exposure assessment

Chemicals may be harmful to human health due to their innate physical or toxicological effects. Physical hazards from chemicals include flammability, reactivity, whether they are explosive, or their ability to cause burns or corrosive effects. These are essentially acute hazards whereby the effect manifests itself as physical damage immediately upon exposure to the hazard.

Toxicological effects relate to the potential for a chemical to cause harmful health effects by biochemical methods, i.e. damaging or disrupting normal biological functions, and include effects such as toxicity (poisoning), irritancy, and carcinogenicity. Again, these may be immediate (acute) effects, such as ill-health from exposure to high levels of a harmful chemical (for example carbon monoxide poisoning; Health Protection Agency, 2011), or they may occur over time from repeated exposure to a chemical at lower levels (for example development of central nervous system impairment from repeated exposure to mercury via foods or air). This latter example is termed a chronic effect and is common for land contamination.

The types of adverse toxicological effects that can occur from exposure to chemicals can be varied. They can include organ-specific effects such as lung cancers associated with asbestos, whole body effects (systemic effects) such as CNS depression from petroleum hydrocarbons, cancers (carcinogenic and mutagenic effects) such as those reported for certain polycyclic aromatic hydrocarbons, effects upon the unborn child (teratogenic effects) such as those reported for PCBs, developmental effects (birth weight, IQ, fertility) such as those identified for lead, and sensitisation effects (allergic responses) such as those from exposure to nickel.

Whilst hazardous properties of a chemical can be established relatively easily in the laboratory, relating these to actual effects in the environment is far more complex and requires consideration of many factors including other sources of exposure, lifestyle, occupation, socio-economic factors, and so on. In such cases it is necessary to establish an evidence base of studies of similar 'real' situations. In the case of physical and to some extent acute effects, the evidence base is relatively robust, for example flammable and explosive chemicals entering properties can result in catastrophic effects, such as those witnessed at Loscoe (NHBC, 2007). Case Study 6.2 demonstrates the potential acute effects of land contamination, in this case cyanide contamination.

The evidence base linking ill-health with land contamination is less defined than for air or water contamination. That said, there is evidence that where exposure occurs, contaminants in soil can present a risk to health. For example, high levels of lead in soil have long been associated with elevated levels of lead in blood (see Case Study 6.4) (Baghurst et al., 1992; Lalor et al., 2001; Maynard et al., 2003; Von Linden et al., 2003). Several studies have also shown that seasonal increases in children's blood lead levels relate, in part, to exposure via activity, with summer days of outdoor play and open windows and doors leading to increased exposure to contaminated soils (Kemp et al., 2007; Laidlaw et al., 2005; Yin et al., 2000).

There has been much concern about reported associations between land contamination (mainly landfill sites) and adverse reproductive outcomes and various cancers. These serious diseases are relatively rare and the evidence of a link with environmental pollution such as land contamination is often inconsistent or contradictory. Currently the evidence base around land contamination is insufficient to demonstrate cause and effect. Where associations are reported, they tend to centre on possible reproductive effects such as congenital malformations or low birth weight, and the better quality studies tend to show either small or no effects. The current state of knowledge is insufficient to quantitatively estimate overall impacts, if any, of land contamination on human health. However, such concerns can arouse great public concern. Furthermore, negative perceptions of the environment can have an impact on general physical and mental health. For example, property blight as a result of actual or even perceived contamination can cause financial hardship and stress and anxiety, which can have a major effect on health.

Case Study 6.4: Bunker Hill, Idaho, USA (Sheldrake and Stifelman, 2003; von Linden et al., 2003)

A century of mining and smelting of metal ores including lead, cadmium, and copper in Shoshone County, Idaho, resulted in high concentrations of metals, including lead, in soils in an area defined as the Bunker Hill Superfund Site (Superfund is an environmental programme in the USA that addresses and remediates abandoned hazardous waste sites). This area, named after the former industrial complex of the Bunker Hill Company lead and zinc mine, covers approximately 5400 ha of the Silver Valley and the cities of Kellogg, Wardner, Smelterville, and Pinehurst.

Extensive blood monitoring of the communities in the affected areas, especially of children, found elevated levels of lead. In 1983, blood sampling indicated that over 80 per cent of the children, including those born since the 1981 smelter closure, had blood lead levels of 10 micrograms per decilitre (10 µg dL^{-1}) or more. There was a particularly strong correlation between high blood lead levels in children and levels of lead in soils in back gardens. Soil ingestion was considered a primary exposure pathway. Remediation of the area, including the replacing of contaminated soil with clean soil in residential gardens, has been effective in reducing blood lead levels in children.

Lead can cause a range of toxic effects. Studies in children have reported neurobehavioural effects in children at a blood lead level of <10 µg dL^{-1} and several studies have been carried out to investigate the correlation between behaviour and intelligence and lead exposure in children. Overall, most studies reported an inverse association between blood lead levels and IQ and that there is no clear threshold for the neurodevelopmental effects in children.

Routes of exposure

Ingestion

This includes direct ingestion of contaminants in soils or via dust tracked back to properties from a site. For residential areas, this is the most important route of exposure. Soil may be ingested directly, either deliberately or from accidental hand to mouth ingestion. Those at greatest risk tend to be young children, who may deliberately eat soil, for example pica, or consume it by accidental ingestion during their play activities. Such mouthing behaviour declines with age. People who have frequent contact with soil, such as gardeners, will also tend to ingest more soil and behaviours that involve frequent hand to mouth contact, such as smoking, can also lead to higher soil ingestion rates.

Exposure models, such as CLEA, that are used in risk assessments can estimate ingestion rates for both deliberate and accidental soil ingestion based upon available evidence from studies of behaviour. Ingestion will also consider indirect sources, for example contaminants attached to or taken up by crops and vegetables grown within the investigation site. Again, the exposure model will estimate ingestion rates for various types of crops, based upon survey data, and will calculate theoretical uptake of contaminants by crops and theoretical soil adsorption factors.

Dermal contact

The assessment of exposure by dermal contact will estimate a time spent in contact with soils or tracked-back materials and how these will adhere to skin. Exposure models will also make assumptions on how contaminants will diffuse from the skin into the body. Again, these assumptions are evidence-based using data from behavioural studies and empirical data. Where data on dermal toxicity are unavailable, this element will often be assessed against an oral HCV.

Inhalation

Inhalation exposure considers direct inhalation of airborne contaminants either as vapours or as particulates (attached to fine dusts suspended in the atmosphere). Vapours and dusts are assessed as those encountered both outdoors and indoors, entering buildings from the ground or as re-suspended soils tracked indoors. Exposure is determined using complex algorithms to model the generation and movement of vapours or dusts, combined with data on indoor and outdoor activity and corresponding inhalation rates. Other factors such as the type and age of the building will also be important in assessing risk.

The previous sections describe the typical routes of exposure used to determine risks from soil contaminants. Full details of how these are derived and applied using the CLEA model are provided in supporting literature published by the EA (Environment Agency, 2009c).

Despite the detailed approach adopted by risk assessment models, their accuracy in assessing exposure relies heavily upon how they reflect the true conditions at the test site; for example, the characteristics and behaviour of site users, residents, or occupants may not reflect those in the generic model used. Likewise the site itself may not fall perfectly within the scenarios defined in models.

Unusual exposure routes

Whilst land contamination risk assessments will typically focus on 'traditional' routes of exposure, such as soil ingestion in back gardens or allotments, the variable nature of land contamination sites will often give rise to unusual exposure scenarios. Some examples of unusual exposure scenarios include:

- particular sporting activities on open ground, for example modelled scenarios may not consider extended periods of high exposure (see Case Study 6.5)
- guerrilla gardening or unauthorised grazing on wasteland or open ground; not considered as a typical activity, but one that is known to occur
- exposure to vapours from groundwater
- permeation of drinking water pipes by volatile organic compounds and other hydrocarbons present in the soil
- exposure via bathing in inland water bodies, showers, and baths; only considered in certain exposure models
- changes to properties from deliberate or accidental actions, for example changes to an activity may have indirect effects on adjacent receptors (see Case Study 6.6).

All of these factors can influence the level of exposure (positively or negatively) compared to the generic model and need to be considered when undertaking assessments. In addition, other factors may also mitigate exposure in comparison to that determined using generic models.

Mitigating factors

Risk assessment tends to assume that all of the chemical to which an individual is exposed will be taken up into the body and reach those parts where it can cause damage. In reality this is not the case. For example, not all of the particles inhaled by an individual will penetrate into the lungs, with many removed by natural body processes and thus posing no risk. Likewise, not all chemicals in ingested soil will be bioavailable, i.e. reach the bloodstream and thus target organs, with much simply passing through the digestive system. As such it is necessary to have some idea of the bioavailability: the fraction of the contaminant in the soil that, through oral ingestion, can enter the systemic circulation of the human body and cause toxic effects (Environment Agency, 2002) of the chemicals.

Similarly, the form that a chemical is in may not make it particularly easy to liberate; for example, it may be geologically bound in rocks that produce little or no dust, or the composition and pH of the soil may bind the chemical tightly and thus reduce its amenability. Other factors such as the presence of organic matter (which can bind contaminants), moisture, and the form of the chemical are also important. Where contaminants adsorb onto soil surfaces they become less mobile and leachable and thereby less potentially bioavailable. For example, phenol compounds are weakly bound by soil organic matter and, as a result, they can migrate into ground or surface water. By contrast, many other organic contaminants such as PAHs and many heavy metals are persistent in soil.

Thus, it is essential to consider these uncertainties in order to assist the decision making process and establish whether land poses a risk to human health. Case Studies 6.5 and 6.6 are intended to illustrate how site-specific factors affect the decision making process and how conditions can vary from those applied to generic exposure models.

Case Study 6.5: Former lead mining complex in the UK

This case study outlines how even in remote rural locations, land contamination can represent a significant public health threat. Historical mining throughout large areas of the UK has resulted in contamination of land by heavy metals. One such area, a former lead mine within a remote forest, was being used for unauthorised recreational activities by off-road bikers. It was a popular attraction and users regularly visited in organised groups. It was evident that site users, mainly children and teenagers, were altering the site topography to make features and jumps out of the lead spoil.

Risk assessment

Investigation involved intrusive sampling at a number of locations to assess potential pollutant linkages. Children using the site were identified as critical receptors and plausible exposure pathways were identified as dermal contact, ingestion of soil, and dust inhalation. Typical lead concentrations found at the site were over 300 times greater than the Soil Guideline Value (450 mg kg^{-1}), with average concentrations in soil where activities took place being 123,450 mg kg^{-1}.

Public health issues

From the data, typical daily soil ingestion (100 mg) with this lead concentration could contain 12.3 mg of lead, compared to the tolerable daily intake (TDI) for lead at the time of 3.6 µg kg^{-1}. It was therefore possible that soil intake from dust inhalation or ingestion of only 1.05 mg on a single visit would exceed the TDI for a child*.

Remediation

The risk assessment concluded that urgent remedial action was required. The scale and location of the pollution meant removal was not an option and, instead, remediation involved securing the site using high visibility fencing with warning signs. A specialist contractor was retained to re-profile the material, effectively levelling the site and thereby removing the attraction for future use.

Lesson identified

Exposure does not always conform to standard scenarios and should be assessed on a site-specific basis.

Since this work was undertaken the SGV for lead was withdrawn and its TDI deemed to be insufficiently protective. As such lead is now considered to be a non-threshold chemical (EFSA, 2010).

Case Study 6.6: Addressing one hazard may lead to another (abandoned copper mine)

Site D was a mine producing many thousands of tonnes of copper ore. Apart from the actual mining of the ore, dissolved copper was recovered by precipitation in settlement ponds. Long since decommissioned, concerns were expressed about the safety of a dam that stored water above ponds at one such abandoned mine, and the threat of flooding to a nearby town. It was therefore decided, on grounds of public safety, to remove the dam with consequent dewatering of the ponds.

The removal of the risk from flooding produced unexpected public health consequences as airborne dust began to deposit on nearby properties. Given the known high levels of lead and arsenic in the sediment, the local authority decided to monitor to establish the levels and composition of dust downwind of the ponds. Core samples of the sediment were also taken for analysis.

In consultation with the Health Protection Agency (now part of Public Health England), it was agreed that a new exposure pathway, and hence pollutant linkage, now existed. As a result, further dust monitoring at specific receptors was undertaken. The results confirmed that exceptionally high levels of dust were being deposited downwind of the settlement ponds.

Remedial options

The local authority reviewed a number of remedial options, including:

- removal of receptors by compulsory purchase
- installation of vertical dust barriers
- covering of all settlement ponds
- excavation of sediments, stabilisation, and disposal
- surface sealing of ponds
- pond saturation.

The final option was chosen as the simplest and most cost effective, involving automated spraying of sediments to maintain surface moisture and hence reduce the potential for fugitive dusts.

Lesson identified

Activities to remedy a problem may give rise to wider implications on- or off-site and need to be considered as part of a holistic design process.

Health studies

Involvement of public health bodies can often assist land contamination investigation. This can be by informing exposure assessments using health studies and biological analysis, or by simple interventions and the provision of health messages.

Health studies can provide useful information to help identify linkages between disease and exposure. Such studies may involve comparison of health data for areas suspected of having a specific environmental hazard with data for similar non-affected areas (descriptive studies), comparing exposures of subjects with a particular disease with similarly matched subjects free of disease (case control studies), or undertaking prospective studies (forward-looking) on matched groups or cohorts to compare the incidence of disease in relation to their exposures.

Whilst such studies can provide useful indicators, there are a range of inherent difficulties in proving causal links to specific exposures. This is principally due to the high number of confounding factors that can affect the health of populations, such as socio-economic factors, lifestyle, occupation, genetic disposition, and so on. All of these add uncertainty when attributing cause to effect. Furthermore, such studies generally provide data *post facto*.

As indicated previously, exposure modelling relies on many assumptions and estimations. As such, there is often merit in obtaining actual measured exposure values from affected individuals. This will typically involve analysing biological samples, termed 'biomarkers' (hair, blood, urine, and so on), for indicators of exposure or effect. Biomarkers of exposure are measurable levels of the parent chemical or closely related metabolite in a given biological medium. Again, there are often uncertainties associated with monitoring for biomarkers of exposure, such as the inability to measure all chemicals, and the often short duration of chemical retention within amenable biological media. However, it is often possible to measure longer-term biomarkers of effect. Biomarkers of effect refer to the measurement of the impact of a chemical on a biological system, such as the liver, reflected by enzyme induction. These are less specific and hence cannot ascribe the effect to a particular chemical exposure.

Current uncertainties

Whilst the processes of quantifying chemical toxicity and exposure from soil are firmly established and well defined, many uncertainties continue to limit our ability to make informed decisions on effects on health from chemicals in soil (and within the environment in general for that matter). Some of the key uncertainties are outlined in this section.

The sheer number of chemicals that do not have sufficient toxicological assessment is a cause of uncertainty, i.e. there are millions of chemicals in the environment and only several hundred SGVs/GAC have been derived in the UK to date. This is essentially a resource issue and has resulted in scientific agencies developing information on chemicals considered to be a priority for land contamination.

HCVs tend to look at individual chemicals, whilst in reality land affected by contamination usually contains many different chemical mixtures with the potential for additive and synergistic effects. There has been some work to evaluate the contribution to hazard from mixtures, for example PAHs (Health Protection Agency, 2010), dioxins, and PCBs (Environment Agency, 2009d); however, this by no means accounts for all of the many and varied chemical cocktails present in contaminated sites.

Latency of effects is another uncertainty when assessing effects of exposure. Some diseases occur many years after exposure. Asbestos is a classic example. Its use is now banned in many countries in view of the health effects that manifested themselves many years after its widespread use.

Finally, in addition to physical and biological effects, land contamination has been identified as a potential source of psychological impacts (Defra, 2009). These can arise from the worry of perceived health risks or land blight, and also from odours, noise, and traffic during investigation and remediation works. These impacts are now being given due regard in current guidance and this will hopefully lead to a better understanding and appreciation of the impact of land contamination.

Risk communication

As mentioned previously, land contamination can be an extremely emotive subject for those directly affected, leading to concerns about health, property value, and liability. Typically, Part 2A sites cause the most concern but remediation of planning projects can also cause concern amongst the local community. The impact of the perceptions of risk to health can be as real as the actual risks posed by contaminated soil (NICOLE, 2004). This can be influenced by the quality and timeliness of the information received, so it is important to provide accurate information that can be supplied promptly in response to enquiries. One of the most important roles for the public health community is the provision of accessible advice and support to those who need it. This advice should deal with both communication of risks to health and provision of trusted advice on risk mitigation.

Risk communication is more than just imparting information on the technical risks; it is a two-way process, and therefore it is important to identify the interested parties. This is not necessarily restricted to people who live immediately near the affected site (SNIFFER, 2010). They can also include:

- the land owner
- locally elected politicians
- those who work in the vicinity
- community groups, including religious centres
- those concerned with any sensitive landmarks
- users of nearby playgrounds
- local businesses, schools, and nursing homes
- local media.

The main contaminated land concerns are about human health, property value, loss of amenity, and financial liability. Therefore, it is important that these issues are considered by the relevant organisations throughout the 'life' of the project. Ideally, a 'frequently asked questions' (FAQ) document addressing these concerns should be produced proactively by the authoritative bodies involved.

In order to reduce anxiety, the public health messages should contain simple steps to follow to reduce the risk of exposure. A site is described by its conceptual model, which identifies who is at risk and how, so health protection measures should also reflect this approach. For example, in a residential setting with gardens, the principal route of exposure is through the ingestion of soil, so the information provided to the occupiers could include the following simple steps:

- good basic hygiene procedures should be followed, including washing of hands thoroughly after working in gardens
- children should be encouraged to wash hands after playing in gardens
- try to minimise carrying soil into the house by changing footwear after working in gardens
- wash and peel any home-grown vegetables before consumption.

Establishing a multi-agency group

As Case Study 6.7 demonstrates, communication cannot be carried out in isolation. In most cases, a multi-disciplinary, multi-agency group will be established to coordinate the risk communication aspects of the remediation. This mirrors well-established arrangements for collaborative working between organisations as part of integrated emergency planning, preparedness, response, and recovery. Members of a multi-agency group may include:

- local authority (environmental health and public health)
- Environment Agency
- public health professionals, for examle experts from Public Health England

- environmental consultants (if appropriate)
- developer (if appropriate).

Once established, the group would meet (either face to face or by teleconference) frequently when works are taking place on the site, so that all agencies get the same information. Local stakeholders should be given the opportunity, through a well-publicised feedback mechanism, to have an input into the discussions of the multi-agency group. An example of multi-agency risk communication is shown in Case Study 6.7.

Case Study 6.7: Contaminated sand gravel pit

Site E is a sand and gravel pit and covers 4 ha. It was used between 1949 and 1963 as an unlicensed landfill, accepting a variety of industrial waste. There was an estimated 150,000 m^3 of waste buried at the site. The site was being redeveloped to accommodate approximately 400 residential properties. In order to ensure that the area was suitable for its future use, the deposited waste was excavated and removed to a licensed landfill; this remediation took approximately 1 year.

Established residential areas bordered three sides of the site. A residential pressure group was formed during the planning phase of the development and health concerns were raised by the residents, mainly linked to odours and dust created during the remediation stage. The environmental consultant carried out on- and off-site air quality monitoring.

Risk communication was very important during the remediation phase, as residents could see that their concerns were being suitably dealt with and that there was no significant risk to their health from the remediation works. A multi-agency group was established to deal with health concerns. The group included the Health Protection Agency (HPA), Primary Care Trust, local authority, Environment Agency, and an environmental consultant (retained by the developer). Outputs included:

- regular updates to the community using a dedicated website managed by the environmental consultant (this included the publication of the monthly air quality reports)
- a 24-hour helpline for residents
- the publication of monthly newsletters on the dedicated website and hand-delivered to the adjacent residential properties
- monthly residents' meetings in the local community centre
- information centre and drop boxes placed at the site entrance, where local residents could visit, mail questions, and directly discuss issues with a member of the project team (local authority and environmental consultant).

The working group held monthly stakeholder meetings that were chaired by the HPA in order to provide a joined-up, multi-agency approach to the remediation work and inform the risk communication strategy.

On completion of the remediation works, the residents' committee congratulated the multi-agency team for their work. One of the key lessons identified was the need to establish a multi-agency working group as early as possible and prior to the start of the remediation work to anticipate and respond to concerns.

Remediation and off-site issues

There is an increasing pressure to reuse land that is contaminated rather than develop greenfield sites such as parks or woodland. Bringing such sites back into sustainable use is referred to as remediation.

Remediation can be considered to be successful when the risks to health and the environment are effectively and sustainably managed. It does not always mean that the soil pollution itself is completely removed, as long as the risks to people and the environment have been properly managed.

Remediation requires the breaking of significant contaminant linkages (the contaminant-pathway-receptor relationship). This can be done by dealing with the contaminant directly (by removal or clean-up), or by either breaking the pathway (introducing a barrier between the contaminant and the receptor, such as a layer of clean soil or a geotextile membrane, or restricting the consumption of fruit and vegetables grown on the site) or removing the potential receptors from the site (rehousing). In complex situations, a combination of all three approaches may be used and the approach will be heavily dependent on the type and severity of the contamination. However, the removal of the receptor (for example relocating people) is rarely used as a remediation option.

Historically, remediation of soil consisted of the removal of the source by 'dig and dump' techniques. This is where the contaminated soil is excavated and removed to landfill, with subsequent 'backfilling' with clean soils. With time, the cost of removing large quantities of contaminated material, the shortage of suitable backfill material, and the drive towards a more sustainable approach has led contractors to consider other on-site remediation solutions. However, improperly managed excavations or on-site clean-up may release emissions of public health significance (see Case Study 6.8).

It is a common misconception that remediation can only result in an environmental improvement. Whilst the remediation of land affected by contamination and associated groundwater is carried out with the intent to improve their condition, the remedial activity itself has the potential to adversely impact on the environment. It is therefore essential that such impacts are controlled, to ensure that remediation does result in environmental and public health improvement.

Case Study 6.8: Former tar works

A bioremediation strategy was implemented to clean up a site previously used for the production of chemicals and solvents for the paint industry, additives for motor fuel, naphthalene for the dye industry, and cresols and phenol for resin. Post-1965, the site was used for the storage and distribution of heavy fuels. The site was contaminated with tar and tar residues.

When remediation began, the local authority received complaints from members of the public of a 'mothball'-like odour. Residents complained of ill-health such as headaches and nausea, later attributed to naphthalene emissions.

In order to investigate the public health significance of the problem, a multi-agency group was set up to consider risk assessment and mitigation. Atmospheric levels of a marker substance (naphthalene) were monitored throughout the remediation process and the results were compared with a Health Criteria Value (HCV) agreed with the Health Protection Agency (now part of Public Health England). The results were fed back to the affected residents. This tar works case study is an example of a reactive response to a problematic remediation project.

Summary

We are all exposed to pollutants in soil through a number of different routes. Therefore, where it presents an unacceptable risk to public health, land contamination needs to be carefully investigated, assessed, and remediated. The required standard for contaminated land remediation in the UK is not to restore land to a pristine (uncontaminated) condition, but to ensure that the land is suitable for its current or proposed use.

As can be seen from the case studies in this chapter, the legislative framework for the determination of contaminated land is complex. This reflects the complex chemical and toxicological aspects of this work.

This chapter includes case studies illustrating how people can be affected during the remediation phase. One of the lessons identified is that a multi-disciplinary, multi-agency approach has often proved beneficial for anticipating, addressing, and communicating risks to members of the public and key stakeholders at the earliest opportunity.

Acknowledgement

We gratefully acknowledge the contribution of Rhys Jones in the section on pollutants and their sources.

References

Baghurst, P. A., Tong, S. L., McMichael, A. J. et al. (1992). Determinants of blood lead concentrations to age 5 years in a birth cohort study of children living in the lead smelting city of Port Pirie and surrounding areas. *Archives of Environmental Health*, **47**, 203–210.

Communities and Local Government (CLG) (2012). *National Planning Policy Framework (NPFF)*. Available at: https://www.gov.uk/government/uploads/system/uploads/attachment_data/file/6077/2116950.pdf [Accessed 29 May 2013].

Defra and Cranfield University (2011). *Green Leaves III. Guidelines for Environmental Risk Assessment and Management*. Available at: https://www.gov.uk/government/uploads/system/uploads/attachment_data/file/69450/pb13670-green-leaves-iii-1111071.pdf [Accessed 29 May 2013].

Defra and Environment Agency (2004). *Model Procedures for the Management of Land Contamination. CLR11*. Available at: http://www.environment-agency.gov.uk/research/planning/33740.aspx [Accessed 29 May 2013].

Defra (2009). *Potential Health Effects of Contaminants in Soil. Report SP1002*. Available at: http://randd.defra.gov.uk/Default.aspx?Menu=Menu&Module=More&Location=None&Completed=0&ProjectID=16185 [Accessed 29 May 2013].

Defra (2011). *Simplification of the Contaminated Land Regime. Impact Assessment*. Available at: http://archive.defra.gov.uk/environment/quality/land/contaminated/documents/contaminated-land-ia.pdf [Accessed 29 May 2013].

Defra (2012). *Environmental Protection Act 1990: Part 2A Contaminated Land Statutory Guidance*. Available at: https://www.gov.uk/government/publications/contaminated-land-statutory-guidance [Accessed 29 May 2013].

EFSA (2010). Scientific opinion on lead in food. *EFSA Journal*, **8**:4, 1570. Available at: http://www.efsa.europa.eu/en/search/doc/1570.pdf [Accessed 2 September 2013].

Environment Agency (2002). *In-vitro Methods for the Measurement of the Oral Bioaccessibility of Selected Metals and Metalloids in Soils: A Critical Review R&D Technical Report P5–062/TR/01*. Available at: http://www.environment-agency.gov.uk/static/documents/Research/P5–062–01-TR.pdf [Accessed 29 May 2013].

Environment Agency (2009a). *Reporting the Evidence. Dealing with contaminated land in England and Wales. A review of progress from 2000–2007 with Part 2A of the Environmental Protection Act, 1990*. Available at: http://cdn.environment-agency.gov.uk/geho0109bpha-e-e.pdf [Accessed 29 May 2013].

Environment Agency (2009b). *Human Health Toxicological Assessment of Contaminants in Soil. Science Report SC050021/SR2*. Available at: http://www.environment-agency.gov.uk/static/documents/Research/TOX_guidance_report_-_final.pdf [Accessed 29 May 2013].

Environment Agency (2009c). *Updated Technical Background to the CLEA model. Science Report SC050021/SR3*. Available at: http://www.environment-agency.gov.uk/static/documents/Research/CLEA_Report_-_final.pdf [Accessed 29 May 2013].

Environment Agency (2009d). *Soil Guideline Values for Dioxins, Furans and Dioxin-like PCBs in Soil. Science Report SC050021/dioxins SGV*. Available at: http://www.environment-agency.gov.uk/static/documents/Research/SCHO0909BQYQ-e-e.pdf [Accessed 29 May 2013].

Health Protection Agency (2009). *An Introduction to Land Contamination for Public Health Professionals*. Available at: http://www.hpa.org.uk/webc/HPAwebFile/HPAweb_C/1242198452810 [Accessed 29 May 2013].

Health Protection Agency (2010). *Contaminated Land Information Sheet—Polycyclic Aromatic Hydrocarbons (PAHs)*. Available at: http://www.hpa.org.uk/Publications/ChemicalsPoisons/LandContamination/ContaminatedLandInformationSheets/1012ContaminatedLandinfosheetPAHs/ [Accessed 29 May 2013].

Johnson, C. C., Ander, E. L., Cave, M. R., and Palumbo-Roe, B. (2012). Normal background concentrations (NBCs) of contaminants in English soils: Final Project Report. BGS. Available at: www.bgs.ac.uk/gbase/NBCDefraProject.html [Accessed 29 May 2013].

Kemp, F. W., Neti, P. V. S. V., Howell, R. W., et al. (2007). Elevated blood lead concentrations and vitamin D deficiency in Winter and Summer in young urban children. *Environmental Health Perspectives*, **115**, 630–635.

Kibble, A. and Russell, D. (2010). Contaminated land and health. In: Ayres, J. G. et al. (Eds) *Environmental Medicine*, pp. 565–573. CRC Press, Boca Raton, Florida, USA.

Laidlaw, M. A. S., Mielke, H. W., Filippelli, G. M., et al. (2005). Seasonality and children's blood lead levels: Developing a predictive model using climatic variables and blood lead data from Indianapolis, Indiana, Syracuse, New York, and New Orleans, Louisiana (USA). *Environmental Health Perspectives*, **113**, 793–800.

Lalor, G., Rattray, R., Vutchkov, M., et. al. (2001). Blood lead levels in Jamaican school children. *Science of the Total Environment*, **269**, 171–181.

Maynard, E., Thomas, R., Simon, D., et al. (2003). An evaluation of recent blood lead levels in Port Pirie, South Australia. *Science of the Total Environment*, **303**, 25–33.

NHBC (2007). *NHBC Guidance on Evaluation of Development Proposals on Sites where Methane and Carbon Dioxide are present*. Available at: http://www.nhbc.co.uk/NHBCPublications/LiteratureLibrary/Technical/filedownload,29440,en.pdf [Accessed 29 May 2013].

NICOLE (2004). *Network for Industrially Contaminated Land in Europe (NICOLE)*. http://www.nicole.org/uploadedfiles/2004-communication-contaminated-land.pdf [Accessed 29 May 2013].

SNIFFER (2010). *Communicating Understanding of Contaminated Land Risks*. Available at: http://www.sniffer.org.uk/files/5513/4183/8005/Communicating_understanding_of_contaminated_land_risks_guidance_UKLQ13.pdf [Accessed 29 May 2013].

Sheldrake, S. and Stifelman, M. (2003). A case study of lead contamination cleanup effectiveness at Bunker Hill. *Science of the Total Environment*, **303**, 105–123.

Von Linden, L., Spalinger, S., Petroysan, V., and Von Braun, M. (2003). Assessing remedial effectiveness through the blood lead:soil/dust relationship at the Bunker Hill Superfund Site in the Silver Valley of Idaho. *Science of the Total Environment*, **303**, 139–170.

Yin, L. M., Rhoads, G. G., and Lioy, P. J. (2000). Seasonal influences on childhood lead exposure. *Environmental Health Perspectives*, **108**, 177–182.

Further Reading

Industry profiles

Available at: http://www.environment-agency.gov.uk/research/planning/33708.aspx [Accessed 29 May 2013].

Toxicity of key contaminants

Compendium of Chemical Hazards: http://www.hpa.org.uk/Topics/ChemicalsAndPoisons/CompendiumOfChemicalHazards/.

Chapter 7

Waste management and public health

Peter Lamb, Yolande Macklin, Andy McParland, and Greg Hodgson

Learning objectives

By the end of this chapter the reader will be able to:
- understand the different types of waste
- understand the main traditional waste management technologies and techniques and their public health implications
- understand new and novel waste treatment technologies and their public health implications
- understand European and UK waste policies, legislation, and planning controls.

Introduction

The purpose of this chapter is to introduce waste management as a concept and explain how the management of wastes may impact on the environment and public health. Many of the most contentious issues public health practitioners may face are related to the potential or perceived risks to health from the management of waste. These range from proposals to build new waste facilities, such as energy-from-waste plants (incinerators), to investigations into the health risks from historical waste management facilities (for example old landfill sites). This chapter describes how the types of waste produced are categorised and explains how the management of waste is controlled.

Why is waste important and a concern for public health?

Waste is an unavoidable part of society and the economy. All human activity results in the generation of waste materials of some sort and the waste produced may have varied characteristics. It may take the form of sewerage waste from residential properties, emissions of carbon dioxide from the burning of coal to generate electricity, or food waste from a restaurant. All of these materials are no longer required or wanted by those who have produced them, and have been discarded.

Waste is defined under European environmental regulations (the Waste Framework Directive (2008/98/EC)) as '... any substance or object which the holder discards or intends or is required to discard' (European Council (EC), 2008). Article 13 of the Directive requires member states to take necessary steps to ensure that waste management is carried out without endangering human health, harming the environment, or causing a nuisance through noise or odours.

In many cases waste holders will have to pay for waste disposal; therefore, a strong regulatory framework is required to control emissions harmful to health, as the lack of economic value of waste suggests that its disposal is unlikely to be managed and controlled to a high standard.

Legislative framework and controls

History of waste legislation in the UK

The need for adequate waste disposal and treatment became increasingly important as the population moved away from rural areas and congregated together in communities. This, along with Britain's Industrial Revolution (1750–1850), led to an increase in domestic and industrial waste production (Williams, 2005). The indiscriminate disposal of waste during this period led to an increasing awareness of the associated public health risk.

To address these issues, in the latter half of the nineteenth century, a series of Nuisance Removal and Disease Prevention Acts were introduced, which gave the local authorities powers to deal with offensive trades and control pollution. This was reinforced by the Public Health Acts of 1875 and 1936, which placed a duty on local authorities to arrange disposal of waste and to control disposal of waste into water, respectively (Hawkins and Shaw, 2004).

Purpose-built municipal waste incinerators were introduced in the late 1870s, and by 1912 there were over 300 in the UK (Van Santen, 1993). Despite this, incineration remained only the second most common route for dealing with waste. The ease of dumping waste material (either legally or illegally) meant that this remained the primary route of disposal.

The first half of the twentieth century saw improvements in the planning and management of landfill sites. However, they had minimum engineering design and, when full, a thin layer of soil was placed across the waste to cap it. There was little regard for the potential environmental issues of leachate and landfill gas emissions (McBean et al., 1995). This resulted in the historical legacy of environmental issues that are still being dealt with today.

In the late 1960s and 1970s, a number of high profile toxic waste dumping incidents highlighted the need for stringent legislation. The most prominent of these incidents was the dumping of drums of sodium cyanide waste in an area used as a children's playground near Nuneaton, Warwickshire, in 1972. Following this, emergency legislation was introduced in the form of the Deposit of Poisonous Waste Act 1972 (Levitt, 1980).

Further legislation was introduced in the form of the Control of Pollution Act 1974, which introduced controlled waste disposal on land through new licensing and monitoring systems for waste disposal facilities. In the late 1980s and 1990s, further UK waste management legislations were introduced to enact EU Directives. This included the Environmental Protection Act 1990, the Environment Act 1995, the Waste Management Licensing Regulations 1994, the Special Waste Regulations 1992, the Pollution Prevention and Control Regulations 2000, and the Landfill Regulations 2002.

Role of the European Union in UK waste management

The EU waste management policy is set out in six (since 1973) Environmental Action Programmes (EAPs). The strategy's focus and approach has evolved from pollution control to pollution prevention. The EAP policy is implemented by the Waste Management Strategy and subsequent legislative measures such as EU Directives, Regulations, and Decisions targeted to specific waste management issues. Key EU Directives and how they are transposed into UK law are discussed in more detail in the following sections.

Waste Framework Directive

The Waste Framework Directive (WFD) in 1975 (75/442/EEC) established the key rules for waste management. The Directive has subsequently been amended several times, the latest of which was in 2008 (2008/98/EC).

The Waste Framework Directive sets out the basic concepts and definitions related to waste management, for example definition of waste, recycling, and recovery. It explains when waste ceases to be waste and becomes a secondary raw material (so-called end-of-waste criteria), and how to distinguish between waste and by-products (European Council, 2008). The Directive also lays down some basic waste management principles and requirements:

- Waste should be managed without endangering human health and harming the environment, and in particular without risk to water, air, soil, plants, or animals.
- Waste should be managed without causing a nuisance through noise or odours.
- Waste should be managed without adversely affecting the countryside or places of special interest.

It also introduces the 'waste hierarchy', which details the priority for waste disposal policy (see Table 7.1). The Directive introduces key concepts such as the *'polluter pays principle'* and the *'extended producer responsibility'*. The 'polluter pays principle' identifies who is liable for the costs of waste disposal or management. It provides for liability to be channelled to the producer, distributors, or holders of a product; this is the *'extended producer responsibility'*.

The Directive also includes two recycling and recovery targets to be achieved by 2020, which are to recycle 50 per cent of waste from households by 2020 and to recover 70 per cent of construction and demolition waste by 2020. The Waste Framework Directive is transposed into UK law through the Waste (England and Wales) Regulations 2011.

Table 7.1 The 'waste hierarchy', adapted from the EU Waste Framework Directive 2008/98/EC

	Stage	Includes
Best option	Prevention	Using less material in design and manufacture.
		Keeping products for longer; reuse.
		Using less hazardous materials.
	Preparing for reuse	Checking, cleaning, repairing, or refurbishing whole items or spare parts.
	Recycling	Turning waste into a new substance or product. Includes composting if it meets quality protocols.
	Other recovery	Includes anaerobic digestion, incineration with energy recovery, gasification and pyrolysis that produce energy (fuels, heat, and power) and materials from waste, some backfilling of land.
Worst option	Disposal	Landfill and incineration without energy recovery.

Source: Data from *Directive 2008/98/EC of the European Parliament and of the Council of 19 November 2008 on waste and repealing certain Directives*, European Council, Copyright © European Union 2008, available from http://eur-lex.europa.eu/LexUriServ/LexUriServ.do?uri=OJ:L:2008:312:0003:0030:EN:PDF.

Landfill Directive

In England and Wales, the requirements of the Council Directive 1999/31/EC on the landfill of waste are applied under the Environmental Permitting (England and Wales) Regulations 2010 (as amended). The Directive's overall objective is to supplement the requirements of the Waste Framework Directive and prevent, or reduce as far as possible, the negative effects of landfilling on the environment, as well as any resultant risk to human health. It seeks to achieve this through specifying technical standards and sets out requirements for the location, management, engineering, closure, and monitoring of landfills. The Directive defines the characteristics of the waste to be landfilled (inert, non-hazardous, and hazardous) and introduces strict controls on the types of waste to be disposed of. This has had the effect of discontinuing the practice of co-disposal (mixing different classes of waste in a single landfill) and of banning from landfill materials such as liquid waste, corrosive, explosive, or flammable materials. hospital and clinical infectious waste, whole used tyres (since 2003), and shredded tyres (from 2006). Waste going to landfill is also required to be pre-treated (including sorting) to encourage recovery and recycling.

In 2003, Council Decision 2003/33/EC was published, establishing criteria and procedures for the acceptance of waste at landfills. As a result, requirements to ensure that waste entering landfill meets the relevant waste acceptance criteria for the class of landfill will reduce the overall amount of waste entering landfill and ensure that waste does not degrade or release contaminants into leachate that might be harmful to the environment. These restrictions serve to protect the local environment (HPA, 2011).

The Landfill Directive supplements the Industrial Emissions Directive (2010/75/EU) by setting a variety of technical standards of operation for landfills. Existing sites were required to provide conditioning plans to demonstrate that they could continue to accept waste in accordance with the Directive requirements. Those that could not had to close.

Industrial Emissions Directive

The Industrial Emissions Directive (IED) (2010/75/EU) requires industrial and agricultural activities with a high pollution potential (as defined in Annex 1 of the Directive, for example energy industries, production and processing of metals, and mineral industry, livestock farming, and so on) to hold a permit. This permit can only be issued if certain environmental conditions are met, so that the companies bear the responsibility for preventing and reducing any pollution they may cause. The importance of ensuring that industries with pollution potential are permitted is highlighted in Case Study 7.1.

Case Study 7.1: Unlicensed waste facility

The environmental regulator became aware of a site that was recycling empty plastic containers. As part of this process the operators were selling the shredded containers to other companies for reuse. The company running the site claimed to be exempt from the permitting process (Environmental Permitting Regulations 2010), as it did not carry out any activities that had the potential to affect the environment or human health. On closer inspection by the regulator, it was evident that the containers being accepted by the company were not empty and waste liquid was being decanted into unbunded pits and other containers within the site. Leakage and strongly solvent-smelling liquid escaping the site boundary were observed.

The site was located in a city centre, near a busy shopping centre, a football stadium, and residential areas. The regulator was concerned that the site could potentially pose a risk to health and the environment. The Fire Service visited the site and expressed concerns about the condition of the site.

The regulator called a multi-agency meeting at which the main public health concerns of the stakeholders were:

- if a fire broke out, there could be public exposure to products of combustion (smoke) generated from unknown substances and materials stored on site, including irritants
- there would be difficulty tackling a fire due to site access issues; this could result in a prolonged incident impacting on local air quality and potentially affecting local residents
- potential for solvent run-off from the site, or contaminated fire run-off in the case of a fire on site
- chemical vapours could be released from the site (for example, by leakage or accidental release of chemicals).

The regulator served a notice on the site that forced the owner to take action to ensure that the site no longer posed a risk. This case study serves to demonstrate the importance of permitting in providing a means of controlling activities and the key role of the regulator and other stakeholders in identifying and managing waste sites that pose a risk to health or the environment.

Waste Incineration Directive

The aim of the Waste Incineration Directive (WID) (2000/76/EC) is to prevent, or limit as far as practicable, negative effects on the environment. This covers pollution by emissions into air, soil, and surface and groundwater, and the resulting risks to human health from the incineration and co-incineration of waste (HPA, 2009). The Directive seeks to achieve a high level of environmental and human health protection by requiring the setting and maintaining of stringent operational conditions, technical requirements, and emission limit values for plants incinerating and co-incinerating waste.

The Directive applies to incineration and co-incineration plants. Co-incineration plants are installations where waste is used as a fuel or is disposed of at a plant where energy generation or production is the main purpose. Plants will only be classified as incineration or co-incineration installations if they burn waste as defined in the Waste Framework Directive. Such wastes include municipal waste, clinical waste, hazardous waste, general waste, and waste-derived fuels.

In England and Wales this Directive is implemented through the Environmental Permitting Regulations 2010 (EPR) (as amended). Typically a permit application for an incinerator will need to demonstrate that the techniques are the Best Available Techniques (BAT), and thus will meet emissions limits specified by WID (EA, 2009).

Incinerators and co-incinerator facilities can cause concern amongst the local community.

Environmental Protection Act 1990

Another important piece of legislation, not directly related to any EU directive, is the Environmental Protection Act 1990, which defines within England, Scotland, and Wales the legal framework for a duty of care for waste. It is a very detailed act that has been amended by various other acts over the years (for example The Environment Act 1995 and Waste (Household Waste Duty of Care) (England and Wales) Regulations 2005).

Of particular importance in relation to waste is Section 34 ('Duty of care, and so on as respects waste'), Part II of the Environmental Protection Act. This states that '... *it shall be the duty of any person who produces, imports, carries, keeps, treats or disposes of controlled waste, or as a broker, has control of such waste, to take all such measures applicable to him in that capacity as are reasonable in the circumstances*' and describes duties to prevent contraventions of environmental protection legislation and the prevention of the escape of waste and illicit transfer.

The Duty of Care is supported by *Waste Management: The Duty of Care—A Code of Practice* (revised March 1996), which provides interpretation of the legislation and practical guidance on its implementation. It has statutory status and, although the obligation is to comply with the Duty of Care rather than the Code, breach of the Code of Practice is admissible as evidence in court. The Duty of Care applies to everyone involved in handling the waste, from the person who produces it to the person who finally disposes of or recovers it. It is the main mechanism used to combat fly tipping, as it requires any producers of waste to take all reasonable measures to ensure that waste leaving their site is dealt with correctly. Such steps include:

- collection/transport of waste by licensed carrier
- transfer to or disposal of waste at a licensed site
- use of transfer notes—documents that include a description of the waste, signed by the person disposing of it and the person taking it away.

Types of waste

The way waste is defined has a major impact on the methods for its management. Wastes are split into categories as illustrated in Figure 7.1. The first spilt is between wastes that are regulated under the EU Waste Framework Directive 2008/98/EC (sometimes referred to as directive waste) (EC, 2008) and those that are not.

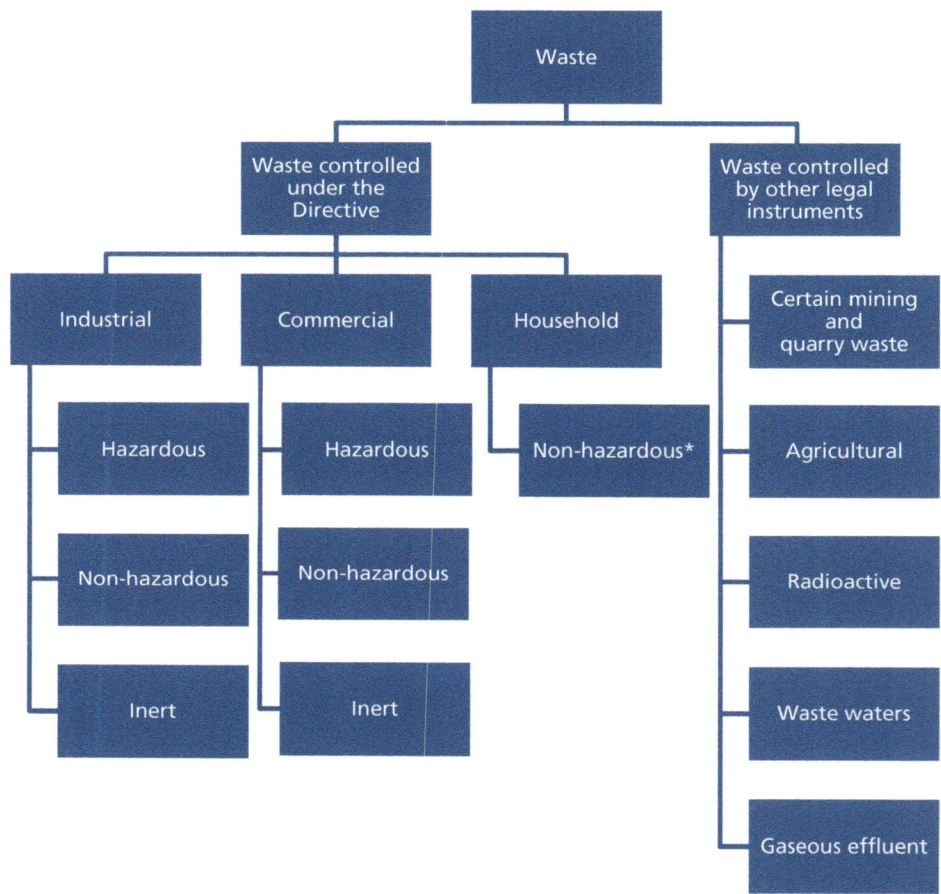

Fig. 7.1 Categories of wastes.

* Municipal waste produced domestically (household waste) is considered non-hazardous waste even when it contains some hazardous wastes (for example batteries, paints, and so on); this excludes those hazardous wastes where separate collection arrangements exist.

Source: Data from *Directive 2008/98/EC of the European Parliament and of the Council of 19 November 2008 on waste and repealing certain Directives*, European Council, Copyright © European Union 2008, available from http://eur-lex.europa.eu/LexUriServ/LexUriServ.do?uri=OJ:L:2008:312:0003:0030:EN:PDF.

Waste excluded from the scope of the EU Waste Framework Directive

Gaseous waste

Gaseous waste is created by many activities and is often emitted directly into the atmosphere. For example, the use of petrol-driven motor vehicles produces gaseous waste in the form of carbon monoxide, carbon dioxide, nitrogen dioxide, and sulphur dioxide. Industrial gaseous waste emissions may have stringent controls depending on the process that generated the gas and the hazards that the gases present to health and the environment as a whole; for example industrial processes regulated under the EPA 1990 (see Chapter 3). Most gaseous wastes are disposed of by being discharged into the air, either directly or via treatment processes to remove or lower the hazard of the waste, for example via a filter to remove particulate matter or a burner to convert toxic compounds into less hazardous gases.

Liquid waste

The management of liquid effluents has similar controls to those placed on gases. The method of disposal is based on the process that created the waste and the hazardous properties of the liquid. Where liquid wastes are water-soluble and do not present a hazard to human health or the environment, they may be allowed to be discharged into watercourses or to groundwater via 'soakaways'.

One of the most ubiquitous liquid wastes not controlled under the Directive is waste water/sewage from domestic and commercial sources. This is predominantly sent for treatment via sewage treatment to reduce the hazards that are presented before it is discharged to watercourses (see Chapter 5). Certain industrial liquid effluents may be similarly discharged to sewer under agreement with the sewage operator. Restrictions are put in place according to the waste properties to prevent fouling of the treatment processes and to ensure that materials that are not broken down or removed by the sewage treatment processes are not discharged, thus contaminating the environment and controlled waters.

Liquids not suitable for discharge to the sewer system are required to undergo special treatment. These include liquid wastes controlled under the Waste Framework Directive, for example water contaminated with hazardous substances and non-water-soluble liquid wastes, such as oils or petroleum products. These substances may be suitable for recycling or more complex water treatment processes, or may be disposed of via other methods, for example by incineration.

Other wastes excluded from the scope of the WFD

These are: unexcavated contaminated land, radioactive materials, faecal matter, straw and other natural non-hazardous material used in farming, certain animal by-products, and waste resulting from prospecting, extraction, treatment, and storage of mineral resources and the working of quarries (EC, 2008).

Waste controlled under the European Waste Framework Directive

Wastes controlled under the European Waste Framework Directive are differentiated into three types in waste management processes: 'hazardous', 'non-hazardous', and 'inert' materials. The Hazardous Waste Directive introduced a catalogue of wastes (the European Waste Catalogue (EWC)) used to identify whether a waste may be hazardous. The EWC is brought into law in England and Wales as the List of Waste (HMSO, 2005); it classifies wastes into three types or entries:

- 'Absolute Entries' are types of waste that are deemed to be hazardous regardless of their exact composition or the concentration of any dangerous substance within them. They include lead acid batteries and fluorescent tubes.
- 'Mirror Entries' are types of waste that have the potential to be either hazardous or non-hazardous depending on whether they contain 'dangerous substances' that present one or more of the hazards shown in Table 7.2; for example, ink and paint when they contain flammable or irritant components.
- 'Non-Hazardous Entries' are types of waste that are not considered to be hazardous regardless of their exact composition or the concentration of any dangerous substance within them, for example, fly ash from the burning of untreated wood (Environment Agency, 2011a).

Hazardous waste

Hazardous waste is essentially waste that has hazardous properties and that, if mismanaged, has the potential to cause greater harm to the environment and human health than non-hazardous waste. Strict controls apply to hazardous waste from the point of its production to its subsequent movement, management, recovery, or disposal. It is defined as commercial and industrial waste that has one or more of the hazardous properties presented in Table 7.2 (EC, 2008). The producer of the waste must assess whether their waste meets this classification.

Waste materials bearing these properties present a clear risk to public health and the environment; consequently the processing of these wastes is highly controlled. Companies generating hazardous wastes must register with the Environment Agency, which keeps a record of the amount generated and how the producer has disposed of the wastes. Producers are required to separate hazardous waste from other waste types. The mixing of hazardous and non-hazardous waste streams to 'dilute' the hazard is prohibited (EC, 2008).

The appropriate disposal route for hazardous waste depends on the characteristics of the waste; it can be treated by physical, chemical, or biological means to reduce the hazardous properties, allowing it to be returned to the environment. For example, the hazard presented by liquid acidic wastes may be reduced chemically by controlled mixing with alkaline waste, thus neutralising and rendering the resultant mixture suitable for further processing and eventual return to the environment. Certain hazardous substances may be suitable for reuse. For example, some solvent wastes can be processed for reuse as secondary fuels in combustion processes, such as cement kilns. Additionally, mixtures of

Table 7.2 Properties of hazardous wastes from the EU Waste Framework Directive 2008/98/EC

Hazard	Waste characteristic
Explosive	Substances and preparations that may explode under the effect of flame or that are more sensitive to shocks or friction than dinitrobenzene.
Oxidising	Substances and preparations that exhibit highly exothermic reactions when in contact with other substances, particularly flammable substances.
Highly flammable	◆ liquid substances and preparations having a flash point below 21°C (including extremely flammable liquids), or ◆ substances and preparations that may become hot and finally catch fire in contact with air at ambient temperature without any application of energy, or ◆ solid substances and preparations that may readily catch fire after brief contact with a source of ignition and that continue to burn or be consumed after removal of the source of ignition, or ◆ gaseous substances and preparations that are flammable in air at normal pressure, or ◆ substances and preparations that, in contact with water or damp air, evolve highly flammable gases in dangerous quantities.
Flammable	Liquid substances and preparations having a flash point equal to or greater than 21°C and less than or equal to 55°C.
Irritant	Non-corrosive substances and preparations that, through immediate, prolonged, or repeated contact with the skin or mucous membrane, can cause inflammation.
Harmful	Substances and preparations that, if they are inhaled or ingested or if they penetrate the skin, may involve limited health risks.
Toxic	Substances and preparations (including very toxic substances and preparations) that, if they are inhaled or ingested or if they penetrate the skin, may involve serious, acute, or chronic health risks and even death.
Carcinogenic	Substances and preparations which, if they are inhaled or ingested or if they penetrate the skin, may induce cancer or increase its incidence.
Corrosive	Substances and preparations that may destroy living tissue on contact.
Infectious	Substances and preparations containing viable microorganisms or their toxins, which are known or reliably believed to cause disease in humans or other living organisms.
Toxic for reproduction	Substances and preparations that, if they are inhaled or ingested or if they penetrate the skin, may induce non-hereditary congenital malformations or increase their incidence.
Mutagenic	Substances and preparations that, if they are inhaled or ingested or if they penetrate the skin, may induce hereditary genetic defects or increase their incidence.
Reactive	Waste that releases toxic or very toxic gases in contact with water, air, or an acid.
Sensitising	Substances and preparations that, if they are inhaled or if they penetrate the skin, are capable of eliciting a reaction of hypersensitisation such that on further exposure to the substance or preparation, characteristic adverse effects are produced.

(continued)

Table 7.2 (continued) Properties of hazardous wastes from the EU Waste Framework Directive 2008/98/EC

Hazard	Waste characteristic
Ecotoxic	Waste that presents or may present immediate or delayed risks for one or more sectors of the environment.
Decomposing	Waste capable by any means, after disposal, of yielding another substance, e.g. a leachate, which possesses any of the characteristics above.

Text extracts reproduced from *Directive 2008/98/EC of the European Parliament and of the Council of 19 November 2008 on waste and repealing certain Directives*, European Council, Copyright © European Union 2008, available from http://eur-lex.europa.eu/LexUriServ/LexUriServ.do?uri=OJ:L:2008:312:0003:0030:EN:PDF. Only European Union legislation printed in the paper edition of the *Official Journal of the European Union* is deemed authentic.

substances, such as water contaminated with used engine oils, may be suitable for physical separation techniques to remove the hazardous oil component from non-hazardous water, reducing the volume of material.

Non-hazardous waste

Non-hazardous waste could be considered a misnomer in that many wastes that are classified as non-hazardous may still present a public health or environmental risk if not managed in a responsible way. Non-hazardous waste includes all other controlled wastes that are not included in the previous section and do not present an acute hazard. This includes many types of waste such as paper, metals, food, textiles, ceramics, bottom ash, glass, plastics, packaging, and mixed wastes such as those generated by street cleaning. Many of these substances may be suitable for reuse, recycling, or other processing to prevent their disposal to landfill or via energy recovery.

Inert waste

Inert waste is a term used to describe waste that does not undergo any significant physical, chemical, or biological transformations (EC, 1999). Inert waste will not dissolve, burn, or otherwise physically or chemically react, biodegrade, or adversely affect other matter with which it comes into contact in a way likely to give rise to environmental pollution or harm human health. The pollutant content of the waste and its leachate must be insignificant and, in particular, leachate must not be eco-toxic or endanger the quality of surface water and/or groundwater. However, very few substances meet these criteria; those most likely to be included are clean waste concrete, bricks, soil, and stones (HMSO, 2002).

Different sources of controlled waste

Controlled waste includes typical waste streams that are generated by households, commercial businesses, and industry. From a public health perspective there is little difference between commercial and industrial wastes as the requirements for their management are similar; however, different arrangements exist for household wastes.

Commercial and Industrial wastes

Commercial and industrial wastes are those produced by businesses rather than households, and include materials ranging from waste paper generated in an office to highly toxic chemical waste from heavy industry. These wastes can be defined as 'hazardous', 'non-hazardous', and 'inert'.

Household/Municipal waste

Household waste is defined by the place of its origin. However, it does not only include material from domestic properties. The 'household' definition also includes waste from penal institutions, places of worship, travellers' sites, and other defined sources (HMSO, 2012).

Household wastes comprise a mixture of many substances that may be used in the home, including food waste, packaging, textiles, glass, garden waste, and substances that present a specific hazard such as household pesticides, batteries, and paints. All mixed municipal waste collected from households is classified as non-hazardous regardless of its composition. However, many waste collection authorities require households to separate materials that present an acute hazard to health from their domestic waste for separate collection and disposal (for example batteries and energy-efficient light-bulbs). Under the new Hazardous Waste List, various household or municipal wastes may be classified as hazardous if they are separately collected.

Household hazardous wastes cover a wide range of materials that occur in the domestic waste stream. These can include:

- gas cylinders
- aerosols
- batteries
- oils
- asbestos
- paints and adhesives
- flammable liquids (for example thinners and solvents)
- garden chemicals (pesticides, and so on)
- household chemicals
- fluorescent tubes, cathode ray tubes, and so on.

Waste management

The key requirement for waste management is that it is done in a controlled and sustainable manner that protects the local population from harmful exposures. The most common definition of sustainable development is that by the Brundtland Commission: 'development that meets the needs of the present without compromising the ability of future generations to meet their own needs'. Managing waste in a manner that minimises toxic impacts on the current and future generations is obviously a crucial part of this (Mohan et al., 2006). The framework called the 'waste hierarchy' is applied to all waste to ensure it is managed in a sustainable way. The hierarchy ranks waste management options according to what is best for the environment and public health. It gives top priority to the prevention of waste in the first place. When waste is created, it gives priority to preparing it for reuse, then recycling, then recovery, and last of all disposal (for example landfill) (Table 7.1).

Prevention

Prevention means measures taken before a substance, material, or product has become waste that reduce:

- the quantity of waste, including the reuse of products or the extension of the life span of products
- the adverse impacts of the waste on the environment and human health
- the content of harmful substances in materials and products (EC, 2008).

Preventing the generation of waste is clearly the best option for the environment and public health. There can be no risk to health from exposure to waste if none is created, and the risk to human health is reduced if producers avoid, wherever possible, the use of hazardous components during the product's manufacture. For example, if a battery manufacturer were to avoid using mercury and instead used alternative, less environmentally harmful materials in their batteries, this could minimise the generation of hazardous waste at the end of the battery's lifecycle. Additionally, efficient manufacturing processes can reduce the amount of waste generated.

Preparing for reuse

'"Preparing for reuse" means checking, cleaning, or repairing recovery operations, by which products or components of products that have become waste are prepared so that they can be reused without any other pre-processing' (EC, 2008). Reuse is preferable to recycling as waste requires less processing and is less likely to result in the production of any potentially harmful emissions to the environment. For example, a person or organisation may hold industrial machinery, clothes, electrical equipment, and furniture that can be repaired or refurbished and then sold or given away to others rather than discarded. This process extends the lifecycle of products and delays or avoids the generation of waste. An example of preparing for reuse is the resale of discarded electronic equipment, such as mobile phones.

Recycling

'"Recycling" means any recovery operation by which waste materials are reprocessed into products, materials, or substances whether for the original or other purposes. It includes the reprocessing of organic material but does not include energy recovery and the reprocessing into materials that are to be used as fuels or for backfilling operations' (EC, 2008), as shown in Case Study 7.2.

If a product is not fit for reuse in its current form, the next best option for its management as a waste is recycling. The recycling process converts used materials into new products, reducing the consumption of natural resources. Recycling is more energy efficient than production from raw materials and directs waste materials away from more environmentally damaging options, such as landfill.

The potential public health impacts from the recycling of waste depend on the nature of the waste being recycled. For example, if not appropriately managed, construction or demolition wastes being crushed for recycling have the potential to generate dusts, which could be inhaled by the local population. Additionally, the recycling of food or garden waste into compost may generate bioaerosols or odours or attract vermin if not handled correctly.

Other recovery

'"Recovery" means any operation, the principal result of which is waste serving a useful purpose by replacing other materials which would otherwise have been used to fulfil a particular function, or waste being prepared to fulfil that function, in the plant or in the wider economy' (EC, 2008). The principal objective of a recovery operation is to ensure that the waste serves a useful purpose by replacing other substances that would have had to be used for that purpose, thereby conserving natural resources. Recovery typically includes the use of residual waste materials as secondary fuels for the generation of energy, such as burning domestic waste in energy-from-waste plants and using solvent waste as cement kiln fuels (see Case Study 7.3).

The use of waste as a secondary fuel for energy generation is a point of much contention but, from a sustainability perspective, it is preferable to disposal methods such as landfilling once all other options in the waste hierarchy have been exhausted (Defra, 2013). The combustion of waste as fuel under controlled conditions leads to the generation of smaller volumes of secondary wastes, the composition of which is dependent on the nature of the waste being burnt and the conditions of the combustion process. Consequently emissions to air from energy-from-waste sites are tightly regulated.

Disposal

'"Disposal" means any operation which is not recovery even where the operation has as a secondary consequence the reclamation of substances or energy' (EC, 2008). Disposal is the least favoured waste management option in the waste hierarchy, as it is the least sustainable and least resource-efficient of the management techniques. Two disposal routes of note are the incineration of waste without energy recovery and the deposit of waste into landfill.

Under the waste hierarchy, incineration is not the preferred disposal route for most wastes. However, for certain materials, such as persistent organic pollutants, high temperature incineration may be the only (and, therefore, the best practicable) disposal route in terms of the protection of the environment and human health (Defra, 2007).

The most common disposal route in the UK is landfill. Landfilling involves the deposition of non-hazardous and hazardous wastes into separate engineered and lined holes (cells) in the ground. These cells are then capped and monitored while the contents of the landfill degrade over time. This process may take many years and lead to the permanent contamination of the landfilled area with waste materials and to the emission of decomposition products, such as landfill gas and leachate.

Overview of contemporary waste management technologies

In addition to established waste management technologies and in a move towards a more sustainable approach to the management of waste in the UK, a number of new waste management and alternative energy utilisation technologies have emerged over recent years. This section provides an overview of these technologies and summarises the potential public health risks.

Modern landfill

Most waste in Great Britain has traditionally been disposed of in landfills, either on the ground (land raise) or in a hole in the ground (landfill). Landfill sites accept wastes from local authorities and industrial/commercial sources for disposal (Environment Agency, 2010a).

Prior to the requirement for landfill sites to be licensed in 1974, local authorities were responsible for regulating their operations (Environment Agency, 2010a). The majority of landfill sites from this era were 'co-disposal' landfills, with all waste types disposed of together in the same space. The underlying principle of disposal of waste into or on the ground was that waste would degrade and its degradation products would disperse into the environment and be diluted.

In England and Wales, the Environment Agency and Natural Resources Wales, respectively, are the main regulators of emissions from active landfill sites and closed sites with environmental permits. The use of landfills for waste disposal in the UK is decreasing, with government policy encouraging the recycling, recovery, and reuse of waste. In 2011, 46.9 million tonnes of waste went to landfill compared to 69 million tonnes in 2006 in England and Wales (EA, 2010b; 2011b).

Modern landfills are subject to strict controls that require sites to be designed and operated to ensure no significant impact on the environment or human health. The Environmental Permitting Regulations set strict criteria on emissions and the management of landfill sites in England and Wales. Older landfills are managed under the Environmental Protection Act 1990, Part 2A (HMSO, 1990).

The main driver for European legislation on landfills is the Landfill Directive (1999) (EC, 1999). Its overall aim is to prevent or reduce, as far as possible, negative effects on the environment (surface water, groundwater, soil, and air) and on human health during the whole lifecycle of the landfill. It introduced three classes of landfill for:

- inert waste
- non-hazardous waste
- hazardous waste.

Landfill sites can generate considerable public concern regarding the potential risks to public health. Common concerns include:

- the waste materials as they are brought onto site, normally in heavy goods vehicles
- emissions (including noise) from this transport and any heavy plant used on site
- waste blown by the wind as it is tipped or deposited at the landfill site
- dust generated from the surface of the landfill and when waste is tipped or unloaded
- the waste materials that have previously been deposited in the landfill site
- any gas generated as the waste breaks down, which is not collected and treated
- any plant used to burn landfill gas, including gas flares or engines
- any leachate produced as the waste breaks down
- discharges from any processes used to treat the leachate
- the presence of vermin and flies.

There have been suggested links to a range of health effects including cancer and birth defects.

However, modern landfills are subject to strict regulatory control that requires sites to be designed and operated such that there is no significant impact on the environment or human health. An assessment of the health risks posed by landfill sites and other forms of waste management was previously published by the Department of Environment, Food and Rural Affairs (Defra), incorporating a review (of the assessment) by the Royal Society (Defra, 2004).

The Health Protection Agency (HPA) (now part of Public Health England) carried out a review of recent research into the suggested links between emissions from landfill sites and effects on health. This review encompassed the results of a number of epidemiological studies and advice sought from the Committee on Toxicity of Chemicals in Food, Consumer Products and the Environment. The study concluded that there was no new evidence to change the previous advice that living close to a well-managed landfill site does not pose a significant risk to human health. However, it is important that research continues to inform the risk of exposure from UK landfill sites.

Concerns about the health effects of landfill sites often stem from historic sites. However, it is not possible to provide definitive advice regarding historic or closed landfill sites that pre-dated waste management regulation in the UK, due to the large variability in wastes that entered these sites, and in their design and operation when open. Where landfills are the subject of local concern, site-specific monitoring and/or modelling is needed to aid any risk assessment and address any uncertainty about the nature of any emissions (HPA, 2011).

Mechanical Biological Treatment

Mechanical Biological Treatment (MBT) is a general term used to describe several processes that combine mechanical and biological techniques to sort and separate municipal solid waste (MSW). MSW feeds include metals, plastics, paper, glass, and organic material. MBT technology has been used for many years, and new MBT facilities are now second- or third-generation technologies.

Mechanical processes include shredding, sieving, and screening for size reduction and separation of components. Separated organic wastes (i.e. food and garden waste) can be used as a feed for composting and anaerobic digestion processes, combustible material can be used to produce a high calorific value solid fuel, and remaining heavy residues can be reused as aggregate.

MBT facilities in the UK offer considerable variability in the scale and treatments used. Process emissions are limited as both the 'mechanical' and 'biological' processes are predominantly undertaken in enclosed buildings and systems. The main process emissions are often associated with the use of recovered fuel in power plants.

Anaerobic digestion

Anaerobic digestion (AD) involves the harnessing of a natural process in which microorganisms break down organic matter in the absence of oxygen into a 'biogas' of carbon dioxide and methane, and a nitrogen-rich liquid residue known as digestate. The biogas can be used as a fuel in combined heat and power plants, burnt to produce heat, or used as a vehicle fuel. The digestate can be spread or injected onto land either as a fertiliser or a soil conditioner.

AD is a tried and tested technology with the size of plants varying from small scale farm operations to large facilities treating sewage sludge or, increasingly, municipal waste. Various technologies are available for AD: wet or dry digestion, mesophilic or thermophilic processes, and single or multi-stage operation. Dry AD uses only minimal sorting and the digestion process utilises waste in its solid form. In the wet process, the waste is first turned into a pulp prior to it being processed.

Mesophilic processes utilise bacteria that grow optimally between 35 and 40°C, whilst thermophilic processes utilise bacteria that can survive at temperatures between 55 and 60°C (Defra, 2011). The advantage of the latter system is that it facilitates a faster gas yield and the higher temperatures help to pasteurise the digestate produced. AD plants can either operate on single- or multi-stage systems. In the former, all the biological processes occur within a single sealed reactor or holding tank, whilst in a multi-stage system different tanks are used to optimise reactions. The feedstock for AD includes a variety of organic matter such as food waste, farm manures and slurries, sewage sludge, and purpose-grown crops.

The actual process of digestion takes place in sealed pre-treatment, anaerobic digestion, and post-treatment tanks and, therefore, there are no point-source emissions to atmosphere from the digestion process. However, where energy recovery facilities exist (i.e. when incorporated with a combined heat and power (CHP) plant) the biogas produced is burnt to produce heat and electricity, resulting in emissions to the atmosphere. These point-source emissions from the combustion of biogas include oxides of nitrogen, oxides of carbon, and small amounts of sulphur dioxide.

Given the nature of the main processes and the controls on emissions to the atmosphere, well-run AD facilities are unlikely to lead to significant human exposure to process emissions. Defra notes that AD provides a means of dealing with organic waste that avoids, by capture and treatment, the emissions that are associated with other forms of organic waste disposal (Defra, 2011). Defra also notes that, provided that the waste put into the process is not chemically contaminated, the health risks from the solid and liquid residues from AD plants should be low and these residues are likely to be suitable as bio-fertiliser for use in farming (Defra, 2011).

Composting

Composting is an aerobic, biological process of degradation of biodegradable organic matter. The end product of this process is compost. Commercial composting can take place in enclosed systems (in-vessel composting), which allows a degree of process control. It can use a wide range of organic waste materials and take place outdoors in open, mechanically aerated windrows or static piles where organic wastes are either actively aerated or turned to promote aeration and decomposition of the material to form compost. Windrow composting may also take place within buildings

Organic materials received at a composting facility will often require pre-processing. This may take the form of shredding, mixing different feedstocks together to improve homogeneity and adjust the carbon-to-nitrogen ratio and/or moisture content, adding water to optimise moisture content, and removing contaminants. Following the composting process, post-processing may take place in order to screen out large particles and blend with other materials (Defra, 2004).

Open-air mechanically turned windrow composting constitutes the main composting technology in the UK. Composting facilities vary greatly in size, location, treatment processes, mitigation measures, and type of site (for example a dedicated composting site or farm, and so on). In the UK in 2006/07, an estimated 3.6 million tonnes of source-segregated waste was composted. Of this total, 82 per cent was MSW, the majority of which was collected at civic amenity sites and through kerbside collections (Smith and Pocock, 2008). By 2011/12, local authorities recycled, composted, or reused 10.7 million tonnes of the waste they collected (Defra, 2012a).

The handling and processing of any form of compost can generate aerosols of microorganisms, which can travel by air (including bacteria, fungi, microbial toxins, allergens, and organic dust). This is typically termed a 'bioaerosol'. Bioaerosols are the main emissions of significance from composting sites. The composition and quantities of a bioaerosol will vary considerably due to factors such as the type and amount of waste being composted, the composting process in use, the level of pre-processing, and mitigation measures in place to reduce bioaerosols. Other emissions include volatile organic compounds (VOC) and particulate matter. There is limited data on particulate matter emissions from composting sites.

There is currently limited research on the risks to health of commercial composting sites. In general, evidence available suggests that emissions from composting sites present a relatively low risk to health for people living nearby (HPA, 2011). A review undertaken by the Institute of Occupational Medicine examined the potential impacts of bioaerosols on people working on, and living around, waste treatment plants (Searl, 2009). The study found that workplace exposure to high levels of bioaerosols was associated with an increased risk of upper and lower respiratory symptoms and chronic respiratory illness. Residential exposure to bioaerosols from domestic storage of organic waste compost was not associated with excess respiratory symptoms but may have been associated with skin disease.

The management of risks from bioaerosols has, to date, been to ensure that dwellings are sufficiently far away from composting sites to ensure that bioaerosol concentrations are reduced to near-background levels. The EA's current permitting arrangements require operators to undertake a site-specific bioaerosol risk assessment (SSBRA) if there are sensitive human receptors (largely refers to dwellings or workplaces) within 250 metres of a composting site. This assessment must demonstrate that bioaerosols can, and will, be maintained at appropriate levels at the sensitive receptors.

Established Thermal Treatment: Incineration

Incineration with energy recovery is a well-established technique for MSW and usually involves the combustion of unprepared (raw or residual) MSW. To allow the combustion to take place, a sufficient quantity of oxygen is required to fully oxidise the fuel (waste). Typically, incineration plant combustion temperatures are in excess of 850°C (Defra, 2013).

Emissions to air from the incineration of MSW include carbon dioxide, sulphur dioxide, nitrogen oxides, particulate matter, and trace substances such as polycyclic aromatic hydrocarbons (PAHs), metals, and dioxins. Any non-combustible materials (for example metals, glass) remain as a solid, known as 'bottom ash', which contains a small amount of residual carbon. Emission limits for specific pollutants are defined in the Waste Incineration Directive (2000/76/EC) and implemented by the Environmental Permitting Regulations. To meet these emissions limits, combustion processes must be correctly controlled and the flue gases cleaned prior to their final release in accordance with the required standards and utilising Best Available Techniques (Defra, 2013).

Concerns about possible effects on health of emissions to air tend to focus on a few well known pollutants: particulate matter, polychlorinated dibenzo-p-dioxins and polychlorinated dibenzo-p-furans (commonly referred to as 'dioxins'), and other carcinogens such as PAHs.

The HPA reviewed research undertaken to examine the suggested links between emissions from municipal waste incinerators and effects on health. While it is not possible to rule out adverse health effects from modern, well regulated municipal waste incinerators with complete certainty, any potential damage to the health of those living close by is likely to be very small, if detectable. This view is based on detailed assessments of the effects of air pollutants on health and on the fact that modern and well managed municipal waste incinerators make only a very small contribution to local concentrations of air pollutants. The Committee on Carcinogenicity of Chemicals in Food, Consumer Products and the

Environment has reviewed recent data and has concluded that there is no need to change its previous advice, namely that any potential risk of cancer due to residency near to municipal waste incinerators is exceedingly low and probably not measurable by the most modern techniques (HPA, 2009).

Advanced Thermal Treatment

Advanced Thermal Treatment (ATT) technologies are primarily those that employ pyrolysis and/or gasification to recover energy from carbon-based components of MSW (for example paper, plastics, and organic materials). The development of pyrolysis and gasification technologies is in its infancy in the UK, but large-scale plants have been built and are in operation in Europe, North America, and Japan.

Pyrolysis is the thermal degradation of a substance in the absence of oxygen. This process requires an external heat source to maintain the temperature required. Typically, temperatures between 300 and 850°C are used during pyrolysis of materials such as MSW. The products produced from pyrolysing materials are solid residues and an energy-rich synthetic gas or 'syngas'. The solid residue (sometimes described as a char) is a combination of non-combustible materials (ash) and carbon.

The gasification process could be regarded as sitting between pyrolysis and conventional incineration in that it involves the partial oxidation of a substance. Oxygen is added but the amounts are not sufficient to allow the fuel to be completely oxidised and complete combustion to occur. The temperatures employed are typically above 650°C. The process is largely exothermic but some heat may be required to initialise and sustain the gasification process. As with pyrolysis, the main products of gasification are syngas and a solid residue of ash and carbon (Defra, 2007).

Syngas is a mixture of gases (combustible constituents include carbon monoxide (CO), hydrogen, methane, and a broad range of other volatile organic compounds (VOCs)). Crude syngas emissions also contain residual tars, chars, and particulate matter associated with the incomplete combustion processes. Larger particles of solids in the thermal treatment reactor are usually discharged as bottom ash and slag. Lighter ash is usually carried in the syngas.

The syngas is typically subjected to a multi-stage gas cleaning process. Firstly, air pollution control (APC) chemicals are added to the syngas to remove acid gases by reaction with sodium bicarbonate or calcium carbonate, and remove volatile metal species by sorbtion to activated carbon. Residual fine particulates and the spent APC chemicals are removed from the gas stream by filtration. Wet chemical scrubbing systems are then used for cooling and the removal of specific gas contaminants, such as hydrogen sulfide.

An emerging technology for syngas cleaning involves the use of a high temperature and intense ultraviolet light plasma arc treatment to produce a 'clean', hydrogen-rich syngas, capable of direct consumption in a gas engine or gas turbine, whilst simultaneously producing vitrified and inert reusable aggregate.

Clean, cooled syngas can supply power generation equipment (through either gas engines or gas turbines). The hot flue gas from these processes is first passed through selective catalytic reduction (SCR) and oxidative catalyst modules to reduce nitrogen oxides (NO_x), residual VOCs, and CO. The flue gas is then cooled through boilers, used to generate further steam for use within the process, or used for power generation or for heat export (Defra, 2007).

At the time of publication there were no full-scale pyrolysis and gasification processes operating in the UK, although a number of small-scale operations were being trialled.

Case Study 7.2: Thermal desorption of waste tar materials

A former large-scale coking works underwent major site redevelopment after lying disused for some years. Approximately 90,000 m^3 of tar waste held in lagoons was scheduled for on-site clean-up and reuse as a sustainable alternative to landfilling. This involved the treatment of the waste in a custom-built thermal desorption unit (TDU), the larger of only two such units in the UK.

Thermal desorption operations began in late 2010. Waste tar was excavated and transported approximately 1 km across the site by dump truck to an open feedstock storage area. From here it was blended in a purpose-built structure before being fed into the adjacent TDU.

The TDU process heated the waste to 600°C in order to vaporise hydrocarbon contaminants. The resulting vapour was heated to 1200°C and passed through flue gas abatement equipment (after cooling), including a high efficiency dust collection system for particulate removal, before being discharged to the atmosphere through a 30 m stack.

This process was issued a Standard Rules Environmental Permit under the Environmental Permitting (England and Wales) Regulations 2010. Continuous emission limits, in line with Waste Incineration Directive (2000/76/EC) requirements, were applied to stack emissions. Ambient trigger levels were also set for a range of airborne pollutants measured at specified off-site locations, which included nearby residential areas.

In March 2011, the onset of warm spring weather led to a large number of odour complaints from local residents. Complaints to the operator, the regulator, and local authorities described a 'creosote' odour, and claims of related headaches and eye, throat, and chest irritations were made. The public perception was that the odour was associated with visible white emissions from the TDU stack.

The Health Protection Agency (HPA) supported an operator/multi-agency group convened to resolve the problem. The operator acted as the single point of contact for concerned residents and public updates were posted on the operator and local authority websites.

The initial HPA response to local health concerns was to advise residents with health symptoms to visit their local General Practitioner (GP) for a health assessment. GPs were briefed by the local Primary Care Trust (PCT) and asked to notify the PCT or HPA of any significant presentations.

An investigation into the odour indicated the source to be volatile hydrocarbons released during the excavation, cross-site transportation, and stockpiling of waste tar prior to treatment. TDU stack emissions were discounted from the investigation when confirmation that they complied with emissions limits was received. The HPA risk-assessed the chemicals identified and quantified through the off-site monitoring of airborne pollutants.

Further air quality characterisation work was requested by the HPA and the operator provided a detailed breakdown of emissions and extended-period monitoring data. No increase in GP presentations was recorded as the work continued throughout 2011.

The HPA confirmed that a comparison of the environmental monitoring data with relevant health-based standards indicated that emissions were very unlikely to cause any health effects within the local population. This advice was issued as a public health message for wider circulation by the operator and local authorities.

In response to the odour concerns, the operator introduced various odour management controls. The excavation face at tar handling areas was minimised, an inert capping material was used to minimise vaporisation, and a fine mist deodorisation system was installed around the site. The operator also launched a series of community road shows to engage concerned residents and issued regular, detailed website updates. The assistance of volunteer odour diarists from within the local community was used to support an assessment of the effectiveness of the introduced control measures. A significant reduction in recorded public health calls and odour complaints was recorded as a result of this operator/multi-agency response.

Whilst the thermal desorption technology was ruled out as being the source of the odour problem, ancillary processes were identified as the cause of odour and public health concern. At the time of writing, work continues at the site. Whilst odour has not been eliminated, a robust public health message supported by monitoring data has been shown to be an effective means of addressing health concerns. The local residents' views of the remediation activities changed in light of the operator's efforts to minimise the odour and explain the process.

Thermal treatment of biomass

The types of biomass that have the potential to provide a reliable source of energy feedstock include (DECC, 2007; SEERAD, 2006):

- the biodegradable fraction of MSW (garden waste, paper, card, food, and wood)
- clean waste wood and virgin wood from forestry and wood processing industries (branches, tops, bark, shavings, chippings, and sawdust)
- agricultural residues and by-products (straw, dry poultry litter, tallow, meat, and bone meal)
- sewage sludge.

A number of waste-to-energy technologies contribute to renewable electricity generation from waste biomass. These include direct combustion, gasification, pyrolysis, and combined heat and power (CHP). CHP systems are used to produce both heat and electricity and consist of the basic heat unit coupled to an electrical generator that is driven by combustion gases or another working fluid. In addition, a growing technology in the UK is the co-firing of fossil fuels with biomass (typically approximately 10 per cent of the feedstock) to produce electricity in WID-compliant power plants.

Biomass is highly oxygenated compared to fossil fuels. Typically dry biomass is composed of approximately 50 per cent carbon by weight, 40 per cent oxygen, and 5 per cent hydrogen. In addition, nitrogen, sulphur, and chlorine can be present in quantities less than 1 per cent, along with trace quantities of minerals such as calcium, potassium, silicon, phosphorus, and sodium (PIE, 2012). The concentrations of these trace elements depend on various factors, including the plant species, the environment the material was grown in, and any contaminants in the soil, water, or air. Chemical composition can also vary between different parts of the plant; for example, higher levels of minerals are found in bark, leading to increased ash production, whereas there is a greater proportion of nitrogen and sulphur in green waste (BEC, 2012).

The principal impacts of biomass combustion systems on air quality relate to the production of carbon dioxide (CO_2), carbon monoxide (CO), particulate matter (PM_{10} and

$PM_{2.5}$), oxides of nitrogen (NO_x), and sulphur dioxide (SO_2) (Jenkins et al., 1998). In comparison to coal, the equivalent use of biomass tends to lead to significant reductions in SO_2, CO, particulate matter, NO_x, and VOCs. Compared to oil, a reduction in SO_2 emissions is observed, but there is an increase in emissions of particulate matter and NO_x. Substitution of natural gas with biomass generally leads to an increase in emissions of all major pollutants (DECC, 2007).

The concentration of sulphur in virgin wood is generally low, significantly lower than in fossil fuels such as coal and oil, and much of the sulphur condenses on the fly ash as sulfates, although a significant portion can be emitted as SO_2 and sulphur trioxide (SO_3). The presence of PAHs in flue gas is indicative of incomplete combustion. Efficient combustion is dependent on temperature and oxygen concentration; therefore, if one of these parameters is not sufficient, PAHs and other unburnt hydrocarbons can be emitted. The use of good quality and appropriate fuel in combination with highly efficient, modern combustion equipment will keep PAH emissions down to very low levels.

Biomass fuels have the potential to become contaminated as a result of being grown on contaminated land or being treated with chemicals, and this may give rise to unwanted emissions. Concentrations of heavy metals in most virgin wood are extremely low; however, wood that has been treated with preservatives or coatings may potentially have higher concentrations (Krook et al., 2004). Consequently, the combustion of treated wood is regulated under the WID.

The chlorine present in wood can react to form minerals such as sodium and potassium chloride or hydrogen chloride and can also result in the production of a number of halogenated compounds. Treated wood may also contain halogenated organic compounds introduced as part of the treatment process. Under specific combustion conditions the relative concentrations of carbon, oxygen, and chlorine can lead to the production of polychlorinated dibenzodioxins (PCDD) and polychlorinated dibenzofurans (PCDF). However, good combustion conditions and equipment design can ensure very low emission levels of these compounds.

Provided that solid ash residues and cooling water are handled and disposed of appropriately, atmospheric emissions remain the only significant route of exposure to people from biomass power plants. As with the incineration of MSW, concerns about possible effects on health of emissions to air are likely to focus on a few well known pollutants: particles, polychlorinated dibenzo-*p*-dioxin and polychlorinated dibenzo-*p*-furans (commonly referred to as 'dioxins'), and other carcinogens such as PAHs. A description of the health effects associated with these pollutants is presented in the HPA's position statement *The Impact on Health of Emissions to Air from Municipal Waste Incinerators* (HPA, 2009).

The comparative impacts on health of different methods of waste disposal have been considered in detail in a report prepared for Defra (Defra, 2004). This report assessed the evidence for the impact of emissions from waste incineration on health and concluded that well managed, modern incinerators are likely to have only a very small effect on health, if detectable at all through modern methods.

Roles and responsibilities

Environmental agencies

The Environment Agency (in England), Natural Resources Wales (in Wales), the Scottish Environmental Protection Agency (in Scotland), and the Northern Ireland Environment Agency (in Northern Ireland) have a key role in regulating waste management activities, including the transport, treatment, and disposal of wastes. Their key responsibilities are:

- **Environmental Permitting Regulations:** issuing, regulating, and ensuring compliance with environmental permits for Part A1 installations (those that are considered to be the more polluting industries).
- **Consultee on planning applications:** supporting local government on decisions on the location and type of waste infrastructure by providing them with data, information, and advice.
- **Waste management:** assisting regional bodies and local government in developing waste plans and strategies that reflect the waste hierarchy and the national waste strategy.
- **Production of guidance:** producing guidance for regulatory compliance and good practice as well as industry-specific guidance to assist with permit applications.
- **Tackling illegal waste activity:** investigating larger-scale incidents of fly-tipping, involving hazardous waste and organised gangs of fly-tippers.
- **Waste carrier licensing:** issuing licenses for individuals/companies who wish to transport, arrange to transport, buy, or sell waste.
- **Data collection:** providing comprehensive monitoring data (in conjunction with local authorities) to enable the amount of waste arising and the final disposal method to be tracked and recorded for each significant waste stream.

Local authorities

Local authorities are responsible for both waste collection and disposal, and related activities such as street cleansing. They have a key role to play in improving waste management in their area, supporting waste reduction, reuse, and recycling, while providing the frequent and reliable collection services that their residents expect (Defra, 2012b).

Where a local authority is unitary (i.e. single-tier and responsible for all local government functions), it is responsible for both waste disposal and collection. However, where it is a two-tier local authority (for example there is both a district and county level) the district or borough-level local authority is responsible for waste collection (waste collection authority), but the county-level local authority will be responsible for waste disposal (waste disposal authority). The waste collection authority passes on the waste to the waste disposal authority that is tasked with the ultimate treatment and disposal of that waste. In addition, the county-level local authorities are responsible for developing and implementing plans to deal with municipal waste, and are responsible for funding the disposal of municipal waste.

In terms of regulatory responsibilities, local authorities will regulate installations with Part A2 and Part B environmental permits (lower-risk installations). This includes ensuring that conditions are placed on the permit to ensure the installation does not have an adverse impact on the environment and human health. The local authority will also ensure compliance with the permit conditions. For two-tier authorities, the district or borough council will be responsible for issuing the permit. Local authorities will also investigate most smaller-scale cases of fly-tipping on publicly owned land, with the exception of those that fall under the Environment Agency's remit, such as those involving large loads, hazardous waste, or organised gangs of fly-tippers.

Public health professionals

Public health professionals, such as (for England) those in Public Health England, provide advice to the Department of Health (DH), Defra, and its agencies on the health effects of chemicals in waste. They provide expert advice to the NHS, regulators, and the public on the public health aspects of waste management. Public health advice is particularly likely to be sought where there are health concerns about emissions from specific sites (for example, see Case Studies 7.2 and 7.3).

Public health professionals also work with key partners to develop evidence-based position statements and reviews. The HPA published a number of documents on waste management, including statements and reviews covering the public health impacts of municipal waste incineration, substitute fuels in cement kilns, and landfill sites (HPA, 2004; 2009; 2011).

Case Study 7.3: Use of alternative fuels for cement production

Cement is made from ground clinker (a compound manufactured from lime and silica with small amounts of alumina and iron oxide) mixed with gypsum. The clinker is produced in rotary kilns operating at extremely high temperatures (approximately 1450°C). Traditionally, fossil fuels such as coal, as well as a limited amount of gas and oil, have been burnt to generate the temperatures needed to produce cement. However, there has been a move in recent years towards the use of waste-derived fuel (WDF). WDFs include waste liquid fuel, tyres, solid recovered fuels, and biofuels.

The benefit of using WDFs is that it helps deal with waste, such as tyres, which under the EU Landfill Directive can no longer be disposed of to landfill. The cement industry is primarily regulated by the Environmental Permitting Regulations 2010, but co-incineration can also fall under the requirements of WID. However, in some areas of the country there has been considerable public concern about the health risks of emissions generated by burning such fuels in cement kilns, particularly given the nature of some of the materials used, the high temperatures involved, and the perception that kilns are being used to burn fuels for which they were not originally designed. Public health concerns have included allegations of cancer clusters and increased rates of birth defects (HPA, 2004). The most common emissions cited as being of concern are particulate emissions, dioxins, and volatile metals such as mercury.

There are several studies that suggest the use of WDF is no more polluting than conventional fuels and, for some key emissions, they are less polluting (Albino et al., 2011). However, there is limited published research on the health impacts of burning WDF.

In response to public concern, the HPA reviewed the available information to assess whether health effects could occur or were occurring. The HPA concluded that '... *if well managed and maintained, cement kilns are efficient and effective processes for burning substitute fuels and there will be little change in the pollution levels in the air that people breathe as this is largely determined by other sources such as traffic. We are unaware of any evidence that burning substitute fuel has caused adverse health effects'* (HPA, 2004).

The Committee on the Medical Effects of Air Pollutants (COMEAP) reviewed available information and published a statement on the use of substitute fuels in cement kilns, concluding that *'no changes in stack emissions were likely to occur that would be of significance for human health'* (COMEAP, 2009).

Risk perception

The public perception of risks to human health from waste treatment and management can vary greatly. Regulators and public health agencies must ensure that their risk communication strategies address perceptions and ensure they are appropriately communicated to the target audience (as illustrated by Case Study 7.4). Not all hazards require comprehensive and detailed assessment. The level of effort put into assessing each should be proportionate to its significance and prioritised through hazard, exposure, and risk assessment.

Managing risk is increasingly central to waste management policy and practice. An essential part of this is open and transparent communication, and understanding and engaging stakeholders, as well as providing balanced information to allow members of the public to make their own decisions.

Case Study 7.4: Public health support to regulators at public meetings

Public health professionals provide specialist environmental public health advice to a range of stakeholders when asked to advise on emissions from existing or proposed new waste treatment and disposal installations, including landfill sites and energy-from-waste installations. Public concern about waste disposal is often heightened due to media attention. Regulators often seek the support of public health professionals and other stakeholders to assist them in communicating the risks to the public from such operations (Bennett et al., 2010).

In addition to publishing their advice on some waste management and disposal activities, public health specialists regularly attend a variety of stakeholder engagement events. Such events include open public meetings, drop-in sessions, pre-booked surgeries, planning committees, and scrutiny committees. Public health specialists must convey clear and authoritative advice at each type of event whilst ensuring the method of communication is specifically tailored to the audience.

With the reduction in landfill capacity across the country, local authorities are increasingly exploring the use of alternative technologies to meet the demands of modern society as part of their overall waste strategies. Therefore, large-scale energy-from-waste installations are being proposed in many large urban areas to enable the centralised collection and disposal of waste that cannot be reused or recycled, with the added benefit of energy recovery. Two such plants were planned for an inner city area. Both locations were locally contentious and the regulator planned to hold drop-in sessions and surgeries for the local residents to air their concerns. The attendance at such meetings of public health professionals, as part of a multi-agency event, provides a focal point for concerned members of the public to ask questions to subject matter experts about possible impacts on their health. The health risks presented by such plants are often misunderstood or taken out of context and this is where public health can add value to such events. Public health specialists are able to provide impartial, local, and contextualised information to the public that is, as far as possible, evidence-based.

Summary

Concerns surrounding the operation of waste management facilities often focus on the potential and perceived risks to human health from emissions to the environment. The nature of the technological and management controls, including those on point source and fugitive emissions, required through the Environmental Permitting regime mean that modern, well managed waste management facilities should be capable of operating without adversely affecting the environment or public health.

There remain, however, widespread public concerns about the potential health effects of waste management processes, particularly within communities living nearby. There is a need to continually review, examine, and advance the scientific evidence on existing and emerging waste technologies, looking in particular at the public health impacts. Public Health England continually reviews the scientific evidence around current and emerging waste technologies to identify gaps in the literature on the health issues associated with waste management activities and the science underpinning them. This process, horizon scanning, is discussed in detail in Chapter 8.

Acknowledgements

Text extracts from *Directive 2008/98/EC of the European Parliament and of the Council of 19 November 2008 on waste and repealing certain Directives,* European Council, Copyright © European Union, http://eur-lex.europa.eu/. Only European Union legislation printed in the paper edition of the *Official Journal of the European Union* is deemed authentic.

References

Albino, V., Dangelico, R. M., Natalicchio, A., and Yazan, D. M. (2011). Alternative energy sources in cement manufacturing: A systematic review of the body of knowledge. Available at: http://nbs.net/wp-content/uploads/NBS-Systematic-Review-Cement-Manufacturing.pdf [Accessed 28 May 2013].

Bennett, P., Calman, K., Curtis, S., and Fischbacher-Smith, D. (2010). 2nd ed. *Risk Communication and Public Health*. Oxford University Press, Oxford.

Biomass Energy Centre (2012). *Emissions*. Available at: http://www.biomassenergycentre.org.uk [Accessed 22 January 2013].

Committee on the Medical Effects on Air Pollutants (2009). *Statement on the Use of Substitute Fuels in Cement Works*. Available at: http://www.dh.gov.uk/prod_consum_dh/groups/dh_digitalassets/@dh/@ab/documents/digitalasset/dh_096819.pdf [Accessed 01 February 2013].

Department for Environment, Food and Rural Affairs (2004). *Review of Environmental and Health Effects of Waste Management: Municipal Solid Waste and Similar Wastes*. Available at: http://www.Defra.gov.uk/publications/files/pb9052a-health-report-040325.pdf [Accessed 22 January 2013].

Department for Environment, Food and Rural Affairs (2007). *New Technologies, Advanced Thermal Treatment of Municipal Solid Waste*. Available at: http://archive.Defra.gov.uk/environment/waste/residual/newtech/documents/att.pdf [Accessed 22 January 2013].

Department for Environment, Food and Rural Affairs (2011). *Anaerobic Digestion Strategy and Action Plan*. Available at: https://www.gov.uk/government/uploads/system/uploads/attachment_data/file/69400/anaerobic-digestion-strat-action-plan.pdf) [Accessed 22 May 2013].

REFERENCES

Department for Environment, Food and Rural Affairs (2012a). Local Authority Collected Waste Management Statistics for England—Final Annual Results 2011/12. Available at: http://www.Defra.gov.uk/statistics/files/mwb201112_statsrelease pdf [Accessed 22 January 2013].

Department for Environment, Food and Rural Affairs (2012b) *Waste and Recycling. Local Authorities*. Available at: http://www.Defra.gov.uk/environment/waste/local-authorities/. [Accessed 01 February 2013].

Department for Environment, Food and Rural Affairs (2013). *Incineration of Municipal Solid Waste*. Available at: https://www.gov.uk/government/uploads/system/uploads/attachment_data/file/181831/pb13892-energy-from-waste.pdf. [Accessed 22 May 2013].

Department of Energy and Climate Change (DECC) (2007). *UK Biomass Strategy*. Available at: http://www.decc.gov.uk/assets/decc/what%20we%20do/uk%20energy%20supply/energy%20mix/renewable%20energy/explained/bioenergy/policy_strat/1_20091021164854_e_@@_ukbiomassstrategy.pdf [Accessed 22 January 2013].

Environment Agency (2009). *How to Comply with your Environmental Permit (Version 5)*. Available at: http://cdn.environment-agency.gov.uk/geho0812bust-e-e.pdf [Accessed 28 May 2013].

Environment Agency (2010a). *Landfills Factsheet*. Available at: http://www.environment-agency.gov.uk/static/documents/Business/Landfills_factsheet_May_2010.pdf [Accessed 01 March 2013].

Environment Agency (2010b). *Our Corporate Strategy 2010–2015: Waste*. Available at: http://www.environment-agency.gov.uk/static/documents/Research/Waste_Final.pdf [Accessed 04 June 2013].

Environment Agency (2011a). *Interpretation of the Definition and Classification of Hazardous Waste*. Available at: http://publications.environment-agency.gov.uk/pdf/GEHO0411BTRD-e-e.pdf [Accessed 12 March 2013].

Environment Agency (2011b). *Presentation—Waste Management 2011: Key Facts*. Available at: http://a0768b4a8a31e106d8b0-50dc802554eb38a24458b98ff72d550b.r19.cf3.rackcdn.com/LIT7382_2bd301.pdf [Accessed 04 June 2013].

European Council (1999). *Council Directive 1999/31/EC of 26 April 1999 on the Landfill of Waste*. Available at: http://eur-lex.europa.eu/LexUriServ/LexUriServ.do?uri=CELEX:31999L0031:EN:HTML [Accessed 12 March 2013].

European Council (2008). Directive 2008/98/EC of the European Parliament and of the Council of 19 November 2008 on Waste and Repealing certain Directives. Available at: http://eur-lex.europa.eu/LexUriServ/LexUriServ.do?uri=OJ:L:2008:312:0003:0030:EN:PDF [Accessed 12 March 2013].

Hawkins, R. and Shaw, H. (2004). *The Practical Guide to Waste Management Law*. Thomas Telford Publishing, London.

Health Protection Agency (2004). *Substitute Fuels in Cement Kilns*. Available at: http://www.hpa.org.uk/webc/HPAwebFile/HPAweb_C/1194947380849 [Accessed 01 February 2013].

Health Protection Agency (2009). *The Impact on Health of Emissions to Air from Municipal Waste Incinerators*. Available at: http://www.hpa.org.uk/webc/HPAwebFile/HPAweb_C/1251473372218 [Accessed 01 February 2013].

Health Protection Agency (2011). *Impact on Health of Emissions from Landfill Sites*. Available at: http://www.hpa.org.uk/webc/HPAwebFile/HPAweb_C/1309969974126 [Accessed 28 May 2013].

HMSO (1990). Environmental Protection Act 1990. *c 43*.

HMSO (2002). Landfill (England and Wales) Regulations 2002. *1559*.

HMSO (2005). List of Wastes (England) Regulations 2005. *895*.

HMSO (2012). Controlled Waste (England and Wales) Regulations 2012. *811*.

Jenkins, B. M., Baxter, L. L., Miles Jr., T. R., and Miles, T. R. (1998). Combustion properties of biomass. *Fuel Processing Technology*, **54**, 17–46.

Krook, J., Mårtensson, A., and Eklund, M. (2004). Metal contamination in recovered waste wood used as energy source in Sweden. *Resources, Conservation and Recycling*, **41**, 1–14.

Levitt, R. (1980). *Implementing Public Policy*. Croom Helm Ltd, London.

McBean, E., Rovers, F., and Farquhar, G. (1995). *Solid Waste Landfill Engineering and Design*. Prentice-Hall Publishing Co. Inc., Englewood Cliffs, New Jersey.

Mohan, R., Spiby, J., Leonardi, G. S., Robins, A., and Jefferis, S. (2006). Sustainable waste management in the UK: The public health role. *Public Health*, **120**, 908–914.

PHYDADES Intelligent Energy (2012). *Biodat International Database of Solid Biofuels*. Available at: http://www.phydades.info/ [Accessed 10 January 2013].

Scottish Executive Environmental and Rural Affairs Department (2006). Review of Greenhouse Gas Life Cycle Emissions, Air Pollution Impacts and Economics of Biomass Production and Consumption in Scotland. Available at: http://www.scotland.gov.uk/Resource/Doc/149415/0039781.pdf [Accessed 28 May 2013].

Searl, A. (2009). Exposure-response Relationships for Bioaerosol Emissions from Waste Treatment Processes. Available at: http://randd.defra.gov.uk/Document.aspx?Document=WR0606_8696_FRP.pdf [Accessed 28 May 2013].

Smith, R., and Pocock, R. (2008). *The State of Composting and Biological Waste Treatment in the UK 2006/07*. Association for Organics Recycling. Available at: http://www.organics-recycling.org.uk/uploads/article1769/The_State_of_Composting_and_Biological_Waste_Treatment_in_the_UK_2006-7.pdf [Accessed 28 May 2013].

Van Santen, A. (1993). *Incineration: Its Role in a Waste Management Strategy for the UK*. Paper presented at the Institute of Wastes Management annual meeting, Torquay, UK.

Williams, P. (2005). 2nd ed. *Waste Treatment and Disposal*. John Wiley and Sons Ltd., London.

Further Reading

European Council (2000). *Directive 2000/76/EC of the European Parliament and of the Council of 4 December 2000 on the incineration of waste*. Available at: http://europa.eu/legislation_summaries/environment/waste_management/l28072_en.htm [Accessed 12 March 2013].

HMSO (1995). Environment Act 1995. c 25.

Chapter 8

Emerging issues

Robie Kamanyire, Graham Urquhart,
and Lorraine Stewart

Learning objectives

By the end of this chapter the reader will be able to:
- understand and explain environmental sustainability
- understand and explain environmental inequalities
- describe and identify environmental indicators for health
- understand the potential impacts of climate change on health
- understand the potential for horizon scanning and the concept of the exposome to identify effective public health interventions
- understand the potential impacts of endocrine disrupting chemicals.

Introduction

It is estimated that a significant part of the total burden of disease in industrialised countries may be attributable to environmental factors such as chemicals in food, air (indoor and outdoor), water, and soil, as well as allergies, housing quality, noise, and sanitation. Human health may be impacted by large-scale and global environmental threats including climate change, stratospheric ozone depletion, the loss of biodiversity, changes in hydrological systems and the supplies of freshwater, land degradation, and stresses on food-producing systems.

Environmental exposures to chemicals are thought to be increasing across the world and potentially affecting public health, with new or emerging risks regularly being identified. Global populations are affected by a number of strategic factors including increasing industrialisation, urban population growth, and non-sustainable consumption of natural resources, as well as longer-term issues such as global climate change and ozone depletion. In countries, regions, or within towns and cities, a lack of pollution control, waste dumping, the use of dangerous substances, and the unsafe use of chemicals will contribute to adverse impacts on the environment and human health.

People are potentially exposed to a wide range of chemicals through water, food, and consumer products. Many of these chemicals can be hazardous to health, especially if they are used inappropriately. Children are considered to be particularly vulnerable to chemical hazards for a variety of reasons but principally due to the rapid development of their organ systems and their inquisitive or naive behaviours, which may lead to larger exposures from hand to mouth activities.

Maintaining a healthy environment is central to increasing quality of life and years of healthy life. Globally, nearly 25 per cent of all deaths and the total disease burden can be attributed to modifiable environmental factors, in their widest context (Prüss-Üstün and Corvalán, 2006). However, creating sustainable, health-promoting environments is challenging and will be dependent on further research to better understand the effects of exposure to environmental hazards on people's health.

The importance of research on improving our understanding of the impacts of the environment on health must not be underestimated. The world is subject to significant technological advances aimed at improving the quality and standard of life; however, these advances may result in unintended consequences in terms of the environment and health, even in situations where measures have been taken to mitigate against such consequences.

There are several millions of chemicals registered and, in the UK, thousands are in common use, and yet less than 1 per cent of these have been subject to a thorough toxicological or health risk assessment. There is a significant potential for many of these chemicals to become dispersed in the environment.

Impacts of the environment on health

The belief that our health is greatly influenced by our physical environment has seen efforts to control and regulate the environment as the primary strand of public health policy throughout the world (Morris et al., 2006). Although the emphasis and priorities may change over time and according to location, an environmental health approach has traditionally been concerned with the protection of population health through identifying, monitoring, and controlling the environmental hazards that produce disease in populations. The approach has existed since the earliest days of the modern public health movement and, by assuring and enhancing the quality of domestic, community, and occupational environments, has greatly extended lifespans and improved the health and wellbeing of communities and individuals. Advances in epidemiology and the biological understanding of disease have further underpinned and strengthened the disease-centred, hazard-focussed approach to environmental health that remains a cornerstone of public health activity (WHO, 2012).

Environmental health threats can generally be divided into 'traditional hazards', which are associated with a lack of development, and the 'modern hazards', which are associated with unsustainable development (Corvalán et al., 1999). Traditional hazards are related to poverty and insufficient development, such as lack of access to safe drinking water, inadequate basic sanitation, food contamination pathogens, indoor air pollution from cooking and heating using biomass fuel or coal, inadequate solid waste disposal, and natural disasters (for example floods, droughts, and earthquakes). Modern hazards are related to rapid development lacking health and environmental safeguards and to unsustainable consumption of natural resources. These hazards include air and water pollution from populated areas, industry, and intensive agriculture, solid and hazardous waste accumulation, deforestation, land degradation, and other major ecological change at local and regional level, climate change, stratospheric ozone depletion, and transboundary pollution (Corvalán et al., 1999).

Assessing the threat posed by many 'modern' environmental health hazards can be challenging, as any adverse health effects may not occur for a prolonged period of time. A chemical released into the environment may not result in human exposure (for example the food chain) for months or years, and even then may take decades to cause a noticeable impact on public health. Similarly, environmental change caused by human activities that occurs over several decades, such as stratospheric ozone depletion due to chlorofluorocarbon emissions or the impacts of climate change, may undermine the life-supporting functions of the Earth. Therefore, for modem environmental health hazards, understanding the often complex environmental pathways through which the hazards move is particularly important (Corvalán et al., 1999).

Traditional and modern environmental hazards are often closely interlinked with socio-economic factors. Therefore, there is often no clear way to describe the development-environment-health relationship that reveals the important interactions and possible entry points for public health actions. Several descriptions of the environmental health causal pathway have been proposed (Corvalán et al., 1999).

A number of frameworks have been developed to recognise the links between development, environment, and human health and the need for specific actions. The DPSEEA model (Drivers, Pressures, State, Exposure, Effect, Actions) illustrated in Figure 8.1, originally a framework for the development of an environmental information system, provides a simple illustration of the way in which the environment influences health and how an environmental state may be influenced by other causes (Morris et al., 2006).

The DPSEEA framework recognises that, although exposure to a pollutant or other environmentally mediated health hazard may cause immediate ill-health, there may be numerous drivers and pressures that precede any exposure and subsequent effect. The network of connections within the framework can be used to identify cause-effect pathways or trees. An assessment may consider the potential multiple health impacts of a single strategic driver such as transport policy and effects on vehicle-related injuries and air and noise pollution. Similarly, in reverse, it is possible to analyse the potential multiple causes of a single health effect, such as lead poisoning in children, which may be affected by poverty and housing conditions, with the aim of identifying the most effective point of control of the hazard (Corvalán et al., 1999).

The urgent need for information on the health impacts attributable to environmental pollution at local and national levels was highlighted by Corvalán et al. (1999, p.659) so that

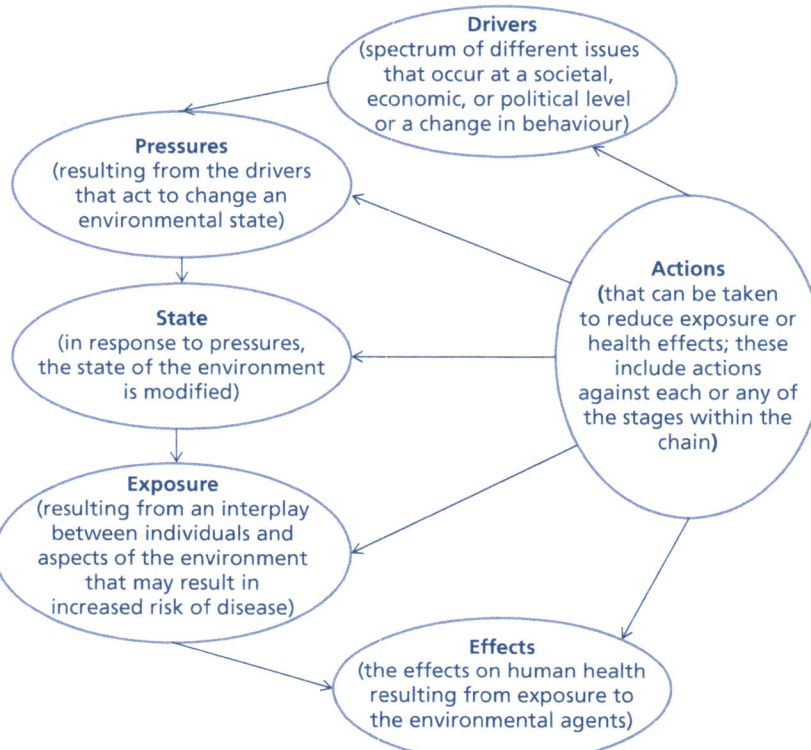

Fig. 8.1 DPSEEA framework.
Reprinted from *Public Health*, Volume 120, Issue 10, Morris, G. P. et al, Getting strategic about the environment and health, pp. 889–903, Copyright © 2006, with permission from Elsevier, http://www.sciencedirect.com/science/journal/00333506.

the implications of environmental health decisions can be assessed, the potential effects of different decisions and choices compared, and irreversible and costly health and environmental damage prevented. Morris et al. (2006, p.902) highlighted the importance of building the evidence base and improving the fragmented and poor information systems.

Global burden of disease

Considerable research is still needed to identify the real burden of disease due to environmental hazards. There are minimal data that identify and quantify the links between environmental hazards and ill-health, particularly regarding their cumulative effect and long-term impact. There are difficulties in identifying the causes or associations behind illnesses such as cancer, which may have links to exposure to environmental hazards much earlier in life (HPA, 2005).

The Global Burden of Disease Study 2010 (GBD 2010; Horton, 2012) was a systematic attempt to describe the global distribution and causes of a wide array of major diseases, injuries, and health risk factors. The results indicated that infectious diseases, maternal and child illness, and malnutrition now cause fewer deaths and less illness than they did 20 years ago. However, non-communicable diseases such as cancer and heart disease are becoming the dominant causes of death and disability worldwide, with more young and middle-aged adults suffering from these diseases. Heart disease and stroke accounted for one in four deaths, with diabetes also accounting for over a million deaths globally. Blood pressure is identified as the biggest global risk factor for disease, followed by tobacco, alcohol, and poor diet (Horton, 2012). Furthermore, young adults are emerging as a new and neglected priority in global health (Institute for Health Metrics and Evaluation, 2013).

GBD 2010 also highlighted disability due to mental health disorders, substance misuse, musculoskeletal disease, diabetes, chronic respiratory disease, anaemia, and loss of vision and hearing. Disability from disease and injury will become an increasingly important issue for all health systems. Greater numbers of people will be spending more years of their lives with more illnesses (Horton, 2012).

GBD 2010 used a number of metrics to record or visualize the results for health loss related to specific causes of disease and injury. The GBD 2010 used disability-adjusted life years (DALYs) to quantify the number of years of life lost as a result of both premature death and disability. This measure is used alongside other metrics, including years of life lost due to premature mortality (YLLs) and years lived with disability (YLDs). DALYs combine information on the quality and length of life. They give an indication of the (potential) number of healthy life years lost in a population due to premature mortality or morbidity, the latter being weighted for the severity of the disorder (Murray et al., 2013). The leading diseases and injuries and the leading risk factors identified in GBD 2010 are highlighted in Figure 8.2.

The extent to which environmental hazards contribute to disease and ill-health such as cancer and heart disease, and how the risks are affected by underlying social and economic factors, requires further research. The health impacts of environmental stressors are potentially wide-ranging, from relatively minor nuisance and psychological effects to effects on morbidity such as asthma, cardiovascular diseases, cancer, and premature mortality. There is considerable variability in the severity, duration, and magnitude of any adverse health impacts, which makes it difficult to compare different (environmental) health effects and set priorities in health policies or research programmes. However, attempts have been made to estimate the environmentally attributable burden of disease, focussing on health outcomes for which there is strong evidence of an association with pollutants (Hanninen and Knol, 2011).

The GBD 2010 assessed a range of environmental factors including air pollution, residential radon, and lead exposure. The joint effects of air pollution were assessed as large. Household air pollution from solid fuels accounted for 3.5 million (2.7–4.4 million) deaths and 4.5 per cent (3.4–5.3 per cent) of global DALYs in 2010 and ambient particulate matter pollution accounted for 3.1 million (2.7–3.5 million) deaths and 3.1 per cent (2.7–3.4 per cent) of global DALYs (Lim et al., 2012).

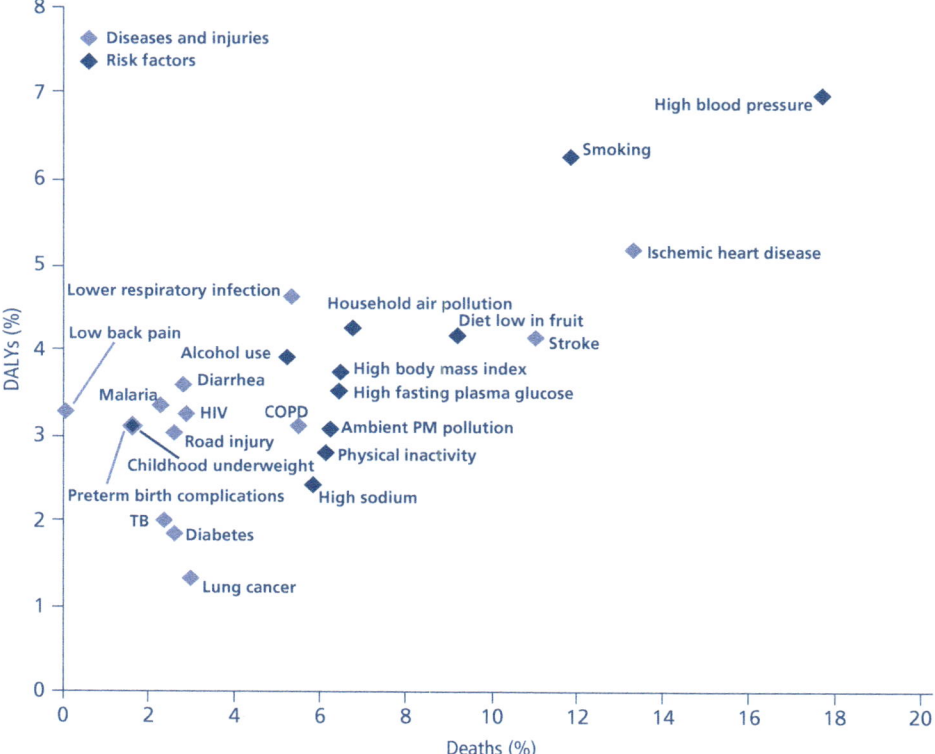

Fig. 8.2 The ten leading causes of disease and injury and ten leading risk factors based on percentage of global deaths and disability-adjusted life years (DALYs).
Reproduced with permission from *The Global Burden of Disease: Generating Evidence, Guiding Policy*, Institute for Health Metrics and Evaluation, University of Washington, Copyright © 2013 Institute for Health Metrics and Evaluation, available from http://www.healthmetricsandevaluation.org/sites/default/files/policy_report/2011/GBD_Generating%20Evidence_Guiding%20Policy%20FINAL.pdf.

Attempts have also been made to specifically calculate the burden of disease due to environmental factors in Europe by using DALYs to encompass divergent health effects and quantify and summarise (environmental) health effects in one measure. This can be used for the comparative evaluation of the environmental burden of disease, the evaluation of the effectiveness of environmental policies, the estimation of the accumulation of exposures to environmental factors, and the communication of health risks (Hanninen and Knol, 2011).

The multinational European Burden of Disease in Europe project (EBoDE), covering Belgium, Finland, France, Germany, Italy, and the Netherlands, assessed the environmental burden of disease related to nine selected stressors including benzene, dioxins (including furans and dioxin-like PCBs), non-smokers' exposure to second-hand smoke, formaldehyde, lead, transportation noise (including road, rail, and air traffic), ozone, particulate matter ($PM_{2.5}$), and radon. The stressors were selected based on their public health relevance, potential for high individual risks, public concern, and/or large economic impacts.

The results suggest that 3–7 per cent of the burden of diseasein the participating six countries is associated with the selected nine environmental stressors. Particulate matter (PM) is estimated to be associated with the highest disease burden (6000–10,000 DALYs per million people), followed by second-hand smoke, traffic noise, and radon. However, the authors note that many uncertainties and controversies remain and the results need to be interpreted with caution as they only provide a crude ranking of environmental health impacts.

The World Health Organization (WHO) has also established a programme on quantifying environmental health impacts, which has addressed more than a dozen stressors (Prüss-Üstün and Corvalán, 2006).

Environmental sustainability

It is generally assumed that any country can preserve the environment while maintaining economic growth. However, a degree of commitment is required from all stakeholders, particularly at local level, if sustainable development is to be achieved. Urban development and expansion requires concomitant growth, including road transport, increasing energy demand, and increased waste, which may place severe pressure on the urban environment, human health, and the quality of life in cities. As a result, poor air quality, solid waste, diffuse water pollution, and noise are some of the common environmental problems facing urban areas (UN-Habitat, 2012). The aim of creating a more sustainable economy is increasingly being reflected in EU and UK legislation. However, debate remains over the definition of sustainability and its key components.

Sustainability is often defined as development that meets the needs of the present generation without compromising the ability of future generations to meet their own needs. Environmental sustainability is derived from the concept of sustainable development, which aims to ensure that social and economic development is environmentally sustainable. Sustainability has therefore evolved into a number of divisions: social, economic, and environmental. In simple terms, environmental sustainability seeks to improve human welfare by ensuring that a balance is maintained through protecting the sources of raw materials necessary for human development whilst ensuring that the sinks for human wastes are not exceeded, thereby preventing harm to humans (Goodland, 1995).

The Organisation for Economic Cooperation and Development (OECD) environmental strategy for the first decade of the 21st century outlines four specific criteria for environmental sustainability. These are: regeneration (renewable resources should be used efficiently without exceeding their long-term rates of natural regeneration); substitutability (non-renewable resources should be used efficiently and where possible substituted with renewable resources or other forms of capital); assimilation (releases of hazardous or polluting substances into the environment should not exceed their assimilative capacity); and avoiding irreversibility (Moldan et al., 2012).

The concept of environmental sustainability proposes the need for humans to recognise that the world's natural resources are finite and with limited capacity to support life, which requires the conservation of natural resources to ensure continued development. Similarly, the European Union's sustainable development strategy focusses on key objectives within the environmental realm: climate change and clean energy, sustainable transport, sustainable consumption and production, conservation and management of natural resources, and public health (EU, 2006). The UK sustainable development strategy (Defra, 2005) has broadly accepted the same priorities, namely:

- sustainable consumption and production (i.e. reducing the use of finite natural resources)
- climate change and energy (i.e. using less energy and safer energy sources)
- natural resource protection (i.e. looking after nature)
- environmental enhancement and sustainable communities (i.e. planning the built and natural environments to support healthy and sustainable lifestyles).

The innate links between the sustainable use of finite natural resources and protection of environments have significant implications for health. The interactions and relationships between environmental sustainability and health and wellbeing need greater consideration by public health professionals. The important characteristics of a sustainable society, across the economic, social, and environmental domains (for example well-planned communities with access to green space, nature, biodiversity, and recreation), have co-benefits. This can be achieved by improving physical, psychological, and social wellbeing, especially for vulnerable groups, as well as minimising unnecessary demands on finite natural resources (Griffiths, 2006a).

Griffiths proposed that environmental sustainability should be considered as part of public health programmes and interventions, such as appropriate actions to protect and improve the natural and built environment, as well as to support the reduction of carbon emissions by individuals and households. Such actions may become as legitimate a priority for local health improvement strategies as combating obesity (Griffiths, 2006b).

Sustainable development policies should be focussed on longer-term, broad-spectrum interventions. In many developing countries, tackling poverty and population growth would potentially alleviate land degradation and deforestation, biodiversity loss, soil erosion, food insecurity, and decline in water quality. In developed countries inequalities are also relevant, as sizeable population groups live in relative poverty; however, additional emphasis is needed on reducing unsustainable consumption, curbing the use of non-renewable fuels, and reducing generation of solid wastes. These actions will contribute to minimising pollution, waste generation, and global environmental change. All of these actions would have long-term and sustained beneficial effects on human health.

To implement successful proactive preventive approaches, development policies and planning need a long-term horizon. Environmental sustainability must be integrated fully within the entire multi-disciplinary public health community (Griffiths, 2006b). In addition, health and environment concerns must become an integral part of spatial planning within the framework of sustainable development (Corvalán et al., 1999).

The impacts of climate change usefully illustrate the challenges involved in developing sustainable policies to safeguard against future threats (see Case Study 8.1).

Case Study 8.1: Climate change

The global scientific consensus is that climate change is unequivocal, with high confidence that the net effect of anthropogenic activity since 1750 has been that of warming the planet. Climate is defined as a long-term average of meteorological conditions (i.e. weather) and as such cannot easily be experienced directly. Climate change manifests itself in a change in average conditions as well as changes in climate variability and the frequency and severity of extreme weather events (for example heatwaves, flooding, and cold winters). In a changing climate it is likely that previous extreme records (such as high temperatures) will be more frequently exceeded (Vardoulakis and Heaviside, 2012).

Human-induced climate change is a relatively rapid process, superimposed on other continuing, mostly slower, natural climatic changes. It will extend over many decades, perhaps several centuries. There is both evidence and reasonable presumption that changes in climate over the past several decades have already begun to affect health and survival in various regions of the world. These health impacts occur mostly by exacerbating or extending existing health risks in populations, for example, risks from the spread of various infectious diseases, regional food and water shortages, and social instability (McMichael et al., 2003).

The UK has undertaken a number of assessments of the potential impacts of climate change for a range of sectors. In terms of health, impacts may occur due to higher average temperatures and an increase in the frequency and severity of extreme weather events. In some cases, the effects of climate change may exacerbate, or be exacerbated by, other pressures.

Ecological studies show that current patterns of weather are associated with appreciable adverse health burdens around the world. In general, a U-shaped relationship exists between temperature and the risk of death in a population, with an increased risk when temperatures begin to rise or fall from average values for that country. Very few deaths occur as a direct result of hyperthermia or hypothermia, but rather from temperature effects on disease, especially cardiovascular and respiratory disease. Currently, the UK experiences a large health burden from cold weather, with many thousands of preventable deaths occurring during the winter months each year. Heat-related deaths also pose a significant problem to public health, especially during extreme heatwave periods (Vardoulakis and Heaviside, 2012).

In the UK, temperatures have been increasing by around 0.25°C per decade since the 1960s, summer rainfall has decreased, and winter rainfall has increased. Climate projections indicate that annual mean temperatures will be around 2–5°C higher than present in the UK by 2080. Heatwaves are likely to become more frequent in the future. At present, the health burden due to low temperature exceeds that of high temperature. However, heat-related mortality, which is currently around 2000 premature deaths per year, is projected to increase steeply throughout the 21st century. The increase in the mean heat-related mortality estimates are approximately 66 per cent, 257 per cent, and 535 per cent in the 2020s, 2050s, and 2080s, respectively, compared with the 2000s baseline. In the same period, the mean estimate of cold-related mortality is likely to increase by approximately 3 per cent in the 2020s, and then decrease by 2 per cent in the 2050s and by 12 per cent in the 2080s, compared with the 2000s baseline (Figure 8.3). These projected changes in total heat- and cold-related mortality reflect the pattern of increasing mean daily temperatures in following decades, and also the increasing size of the population in most UK regions during the 21st century.

If the size of the population is kept constant, the nationwide heat-related mortality is projected to increase by approximately 46 per cent, 169 per cent, and 329 per cent in the 2020s, 2050s, and 2080s,

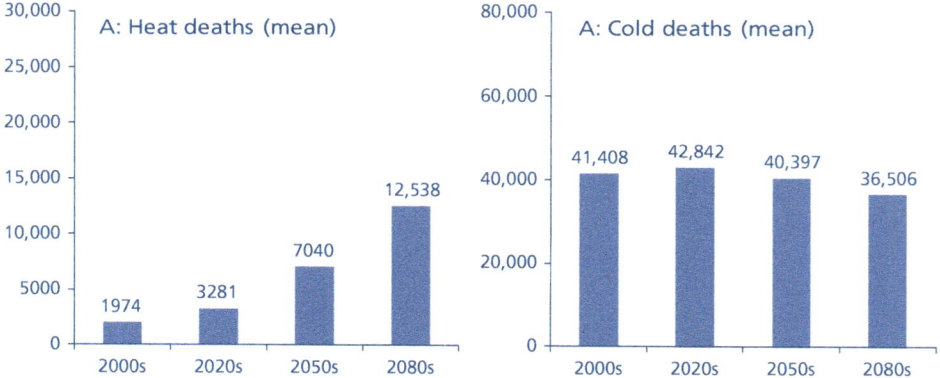

Fig. 8.3 Mean estimates of heat-related and cold-related deaths in the UK per year for all ages based on an ensemble of nine climate model realisations (the additional heatwave effect in London is not included).

Reproduced with permission from Vardoulakis, S. and Heaviside, C. (Eds.), *Health Effects of Climate Change in the UK 2012: Current evidence, recommendations and research gaps*, Centre for Radiation, Chemical and Environmental Hazards, Health Protection Agency, UK, Copyright © 2012, available from http://www.hpa.org.uk/hecc2012.

respectively, while the cold-related mortality is projected to decrease by approximately 9 per cent, 26 per cent, and 40 per cent over the same decades compared with the 2000s baseline (Vardoulakis and Heaviside, 2012).

The *Health Effects of Climate Change in the UK* report (Vardoulakis and Heaviside, 2012) assessed the number of excess deaths due to heat and cold in the UK for four different age groups (0–64, 65–74, 75–84, and over 85 years). Although the relative risks for individual age groups are not statistically significant in all cases, the results indicated that the burden of heat and cold is much larger in the age groups of 75–84 years and, in particular, those over 85 years of age, compared to younger age groups. Heat-related mortality in the age groups over 65 years is expected to increase steeply in the second half of the 21st century, while cold-related mortality will decrease at a lower rate over the same period. Therefore, future health burdens are likely to be amplified by an ageing population (Vardoulakis and Heaviside, 2012).

The report noted that future health impacts of air pollution due to climate change are difficult to project, since air pollution levels are largely controlled by man-made atmospheric emissions of chemicals, as well as weather and climate. The report focussed on ozone, a respiratory irritant that is strongly influenced by the climate, and assessed the future impacts of ground level ozone pollution on health for a range of emission scenarios. Current ozone-related mortality is estimated to be up to 11,900 premature deaths per year in the UK, if no threshold for the effects of ozone is assumed. The report suggests increases in mortality of up to 14,000 to 15,000 for the 2030s, depending on future ozone precursor emissions. An increase in temperature of 5°C is projected to lead to an increased ozone-related health burden of 4 per cent (around 500 premature deaths per year) compared with the baseline and assuming no threshold effect, with the south-east of England seeing the largest increases.

The report notes that assessing the climate change impacts on floods and droughts, aeroallergens, UV radiation, and the indoor environment is challenging. It is thought that changes in seasonality, temperature, and weather patterns in the UK, related to climate change, may have an effect on human exposure to pollen grains, as well as affecting the potency of aeroallergens. Allergic people may suffer from longer pollen seasons and more rapid symptom development. It is likely that climate change will increase river and coastal flood risk in the coming decades. Warmer summers may increase population exposure to UV radiation due to increased time spent outdoors, which could increase health risks associated with UV including some skin cancers. However, moderate exposure to the sun is beneficial for the production of vitamin D. Lifestyle and behaviours will therefore have a strong influence on any impacts of changes to levels of UV radiation. Similarly, the UK population spends 90 per cent of their time indoors, and climate change may exacerbate health risks associated with increased temperatures within buildings, indoor air pollution, or flood damage. Critical infrastructure such as hospitals, health centres, and care homes may be adversely affected during heatwaves or following flooding.

Environmental inequalities

The unequal distribution of health and wellbeing in national populations is a major challenge for public health. This is true for environmental health conditions and the risk of exposure to such conditions, which vary strongly with a range of socio-demographic determinants (WHO, 2012).

In 2008, the final report of the WHO Commission on Social Determinants of Health (CSDH) (WHO, 2008) concluded that inequalities in health are a major challenge for both development and overall progress in countries. Such inequalities also exist within environmental health; almost all countries have some groups of their population at greater risk of experiencing harmful environmental conditions than others (WHO, 2012).

Health inequalities are one of the main challenges for public health throughout Europe. People with lower levels of education, occupation, and/or income tend to die younger and have a higher prevalence of most types of health problems. It is increasingly recognised that exposure to environmental pollutants and differences in the quality and location of residential accommodation are a major contributing factor in health inequalities (Bolte et al., 2010).

Environmental health inequalities can occur through a variety of mechanisms, although they typically involve particular people who are disadvantaged living in areas with a greater concentration of environmental hazards and a lack of positive environmental qualities. For example, there is evidence that there is a tendency for poorer, less educated, disadvantaged people, or ethnic minorities, to live closer to waste treatment facilities. It is also recognised that these individuals may be more susceptible to potential adverse health effects, as the same level of environmental exposure can result in a greater health impact when borne by a disadvantaged population. Any adverse health effects due to proximity to environmental hazards may be compounded by the adverse effects of social disadvantage or underlying ill-health, resulting in a lower ability to respond to the environmental stress (Martuzzi et al., 2010).

The example in Box 8.1 illustrates that marginalised and disadvantaged groups may be disproportionately exposed and vulnerable to environmental risks. In England, people living in the poorest neighbourhoods will, on average, die seven years earlier than people living in the richest. There is also variation in health expectancy, the time period in which they can expect to live in good health, with an average difference in DALYs of 17 years (Marmot, 2010).

> **Box 8.1 Example of the possible ways that marginalised and disadvantaged groups could be disproportionately exposed and vulnerable to environmental risks**
>
> A theoretical illustration considers particular vulnerable groups such as the elderly and those on a low income occupying low-quality housing with associated poorly maintained gas or solid fuel heating systems, resulting in the potential for exposure to carbon monoxide (CO). The elderly, cognitively impaired, and those with limited education may also be less knowledgeable about the hazards of CO, and at greater risk as they tend to remain at home and, in a struggle to keep warm on a limited income, deliberately limit ventilation to save on fuel costs. To further compound the risk, the elderly are typically more vulnerable to the adverse health effects of CO due to pre-existing illness or impaired cardiorespiratory function, thus illustrating that socio-demographic factors may also influence individual vulnerability (WHO, 2012).

Since 2007, the majority of human beings live in urban settings. Globally, urbanisation is reshaping population health problems, particularly among the urban poor, and particularly for non-communicable diseases, accidental and violent injuries, and deaths and impact from ecological disaster (WHO, 2012). The CSDH report recognised that children are particularly vulnerable and that poor children are confronted with widespread environmental inequalities in terms of accumulation of multiple environmental risks. The cumulative risk of environmental exposures can contribute both directly and indirectly to a variety of adverse health outcomes in children (Bolte et al., 2010).

The CSDH report has highlighted the need to develop appropriate measures of environmental quality. There is a requirement for robust indicators to demonstrate the relationship between environmental health risks and different socio-demographic variables and provide an improved understanding of specific risk groups and their exposure. The CSDH called such measures 'indicators of environmental health inequality'. However, indicators have no practical value unless they can be used to gather and process information about environmental health inequalities in practice, and this demands data, which is often lacking (WHO, 2012).

The development of suitable indicators has been taken forward by the WHO (European Centre for Environment and Health in Bonn (WHO ECEH-Bonn)) through the Environment and Health Information Systems (ENHIS), which was developed to address the need for good quality and reliable information on the environment, population health, and their linkages. ENHIS can be used to identify and prioritise issues, and develop and evaluate policies and actions in order to reduce the burden of disease via control of hazardous environmental exposures and their effects. ENHIS developed a methodology for a core set of 26 indicators to monitor and report the health status of a country in relation to environmental risk factors. It was based on the DPSEEA model (Figure 8.1), which allows for the mapping of a wide spectrum of environmental health issues. The indicators address the four regional priority goals (RPGs) to assess the burden of disease attributed to environmental exposures and hazards. The main foci of the four RPGs are: water, sanitation, and health; accidents, injuries, obesity, and physical activity; indoor and outdoor air pollution; and chemical, physical, and biological agents. The information system contains data for many of the 53 member states of the WHO European Region and is available on the Internet (WHO, 2013).

Case Study 8.2: Use of sub-national indicators to improve public health in Europe (UNIPHE)

At the Fifth Ministerial Conference on Environment and Health, which was organised by the WHO in Parma, Italy in 2010, the 53 member states in the WHO European Region set clear targets to reduce the harm to health from environmental exposures within the next decade. The aim of UNIPHE was to provide information for the reduction of the burden of disease from harmful environmental exposures by creating a sustainable, harmonised environment and health information system. The project was co-financed by the European Commission with seven European partners from the UK, Germany, Hungary, Lithuania, Romania, Slovenia, and Spain.

The project built on previous work that used sets of indicators to carry out national assessments of the health status of European populations. The existing indicator sets included the Environment and Health Information System (ENHIS), the European Community Health Indicators Monitoring (ECHIM), and the European Community Health Indicators (ECHI). The aim of these systems was to enable policy makers to undertake rapid comparisons of the performance of their country against others with very little effort. Some policies and interventions have a positive outcome nationally, but it is often necessary to have policies and interventions targeted at sub-populations where a number of similarities may exist, such as access to hospitals or living in close proximity to industrial processes.

Given the usefulness of ENHIS and other systems, it seemed logical to evaluate and develop the use of such a system at a sub-national (regional and/or local) level in Europe. UNIPHE used the core set of ENHIS indicators to assess public health linked to environmental exposures at a regional level. Furthermore, social, cultural, and political issues were also considered through the use of a modified DPSEEA model (Morris et al., 2006). This modified model recognises that whether a particular aspect of the environment (a state) results in an exposure for the individual and whether that exposure results in a health effect (positive or negative) is influenced by context. That context may be demographic, social, behavioural, cultural, or genetic and aspects of context may also be targets for policy and action to improve the health outcome.

The project developed a tool that will quickly enable public health practitioners, policy makers, researchers, and the public to assess the health status of sub-populations within European countries (UNIPHE). It will help to highlight public health issues in sub-populations so that member states can develop and implement appropriate interventions or programmes followed by monitoring for improved health outcomes. The system was built with the capacity to accommodate information from all EU member states and therefore contemporaneous data can be uploaded as and when it becomes available, ensuring the long-term sustainability of the system.

This project should increase knowledge and enable assessment of the effectiveness of interventions through the monitoring of predefined outcomes. The compendium of information is an invaluable tool as it also provides a repository of policies and interventions, available at sub-national level for seven of the core set of indicators. Despite the lack of evidence relating to the effectiveness of implemented policies or interventions, the compendium provides a wealth of information that may be useful to and inspire policy makers and public health professionals in developing health-related policies.

Horizon scanning

Along with the ability to assess current threats and impacts of the environment on health through the development of indicators and metrics (see Case Study 8.2.), there is a need to consider evolving threats and hazards and adopt proactive preventive approaches, through development policies and planning that need a long-time horizon. Many tools have been developed to try to anticipate and take advantage of new developments that become important in the future. Horizon scanning is the fundamental first step in examining potential threats, opportunities, and likely developments, including, but not restricted to, those at the margins of current thinking and planning. It may explore novel and unexpected issues as well as persistent problems or trends. This creates an evidence-based approach to identifying new threats and opportunities, which can complement the more traditional expert-driven identification of new issues.

The aim of horizon scanning in public health is to identify new science, technology, and social developments that will alter population level exposure to hazardous substances. New science might improve the understanding of how a hazardous substance affects health, for example, identifying an effect at lower exposure levels, or linking an exposure to a previously unrecognised health condition. It is also possible to use new scientific discoveries to enhance health where positive impacts are identified, for example from exposure to green space. For any scientific or technical development there will be benefits and costs, and how they materialise will strongly relate to the way in which society treats and utilises them. New technologies can alter public risk in a wide range of situations, for example new industrial developments using new technologies for waste disposal. New technologies can re-introduce well recognised hazards into new situations that might alter risk, for example increased concentration of detergents to reduce packaging in a bid to improve sustainability, or introduce new real or perceived threats, for example home fabrication and associated chemicals not usually found in domestic settings. New technologies can also be used to improve health protection, for example, by measuring personal exposure to pollution, or new methods for cleaning up contaminated areas. Social developments are extremely important in relation to public health risk, but challenging to anticipate. It has been suggested that social factors will be the most important when considering the magnitude of impact from any new development or activity.

One of the main challenges of horizon scanning is developing methods that allow filtering of large volumes of information without specifying key words, as by definition you do not know what you are scanning for, only that it is new and relevant. There are considerable efforts towards developing semantic tools to automate this process, but humans have unique abilities to deal with variation in data that cannot easily be matched using artificial intelligence alone. This concept is illustrated in the Committee for Science and Technology Challenges to US National Security Interests Big Data workshop report (Committee for Science and Technology Challenges to US National Security Interests, 2012), which describes two important computing events related to the chess analogy. This has relevance to creating an effective horizon scanning method, as it requires most importantly a robust process, coupled with computer skills to cope with the volume of data and human skills to deal with the variation and filtering of the data.

The exposome study

The exposome is a relatively new concept that seeks to provide more quantitative data in relation to environmental exposures to stressors, which can be combined with genetic data to help understand overall disease mechanisms and risks. The identification and mapping of the human genome in 2000 was expected to lead to a new era of molecular medicine, providing new ways to prevent, diagnose, treat, and cure disease. Thus far, the benefits of the human genome project have not matched the expectations of major breakthroughs or significant advances such as a reduction in the prevalence of major chronic diseases such as cancer.

In the UK, the Human Genomics Strategy Group published their vision of how genetic information can help to transform healthcare in the future (Human Genomics Strategy Group, 2012). The report includes a focus on public health, suggesting genomics will contribute to the outcomes across all five domains of the draft public health outcomes framework by improving our understanding of gene–environment interactions and the causes of common diseases, enabling people to change health behaviours to reduce their risks.

The exposome is described as representing 'everything a person is exposed to in the environment, that's not in the genes'. That includes stress, diet, lifestyle choices, recreational and medicinal drug use, and infections, to name a few. The big difference is that the exposome changes throughout life as our bodies, diets, and lifestyles change (Hamzelou, 2010).

The concept of exposome was first referenced in 2005 (Wild, 2005). The author raised concerns that a focus on studying associations between genetics and disease had been to the detriment of efforts to improve information on environmental (non-genetic) factors. Therefore, a shift from genetic testing for clinical management of patients towards population level assessment using epidemiological tools might help to identify effective public health measures for reducing chronic disease. The influence of genes on chronic health conditions varies, but often the environmental (non-genetic) influences are far greater.

Wild proposed that more effective public health initiative interventions would be found by shifting the focus towards identifying the 'exposome', and subsequent development of exposure estimates and data processing tools (Wild, 2005). A useful example is the development of exposure biomarkers for infectious disease, compared to the different approaches taken for cancer epidemiology studies into chemical factors. In principle, mRNA, protein, and metabolite expression might contribute to a step change in how exposure can be estimated, but considerable research effort will be required to determine if this is the case. Wild further suggests that exposome estimates might dramatically improve understanding about how environmental risk factors contribute to cancer (Wild, 2011), in combination with other developments such as refinements in personal and environmental monitoring, geographic information systems, and sophisticated questionnaires.

Wild highlighted the global epidemiology of cancer up until 2030, suggesting that the greatest impact may be on developing countries. He called for a more balanced, two-way strategy to translate research into both clinical practice and public health initiatives. In addition, he recommended a global collaborative approach to maximise the advances that can be realised from new exposome developments. Another recent article builds on these previous descriptions to improve how the exposome is defined and consider how its realisation may be achieved in epidemiological studies (Wild, 2012).

New technologies may allow more accurate estimates of exposures to environmental stressors, such as highly sensitive analytical techniques that can measure very low amounts of polycyclic aromatic hydrocarbons or arsenic species (Martyn et al., 2009). The use of protein adduct analysis using chromatography and tandem mass spectrometry has been used to estimate neo-natal exposure to benzene, and the expansion of these tools could create large economic and health benefits. In the past, improved monitoring capability has motivated reductions in exposures (for example lead); this could be similar for exposome advances in the future. Collaborations could be created, using a similar approach to that used to sequence the genome, in order to maximise the impact of exposome research. The role of microbial transformation of toxic chemicals can also be considered using the exposome concept, which may be more important than previously recognised in contributing to environmental health risks (Betts, 2011).

The opportunity for coherence in environmental health research will only be realised by a balanced approach, combining information from external exposures with analysis of biological samples, to reflect internal chemical variations (Lioy and Rappaport, 2011). Some of the difficulties that could arise if information on internal states is not coupled with external factors include capturing effects from complex mixtures and a lack of biological markers for exposure to some hazards, for example noise (Peters et al., 2012). However, the relatively small number of substances studied in relation to long-term human environmental exposures indicates the potential for the development of data processing tools to generate hypotheses on important factors relating to chronic diseases that were previously unrecognised (Rappaport, 2012). A step towards improving the ability to evaluate population-wide exposures may come from making well-curated data sets publically available (Traynor and Singleton, 2010).

The increasing interest in the exposome concept has led to a call for proposals to meet the challenges raised by the concept of the exposome research, and development funding supported jointly by the European Union Horizon 2020 research programme and the National Institute of Environmental Health Sciences in the USA (Birnbaum, 2010).

The literature focusses on specific chemicals, which may be one component of the total exposome, including interesting examples of how different types of data and models can be used to contribute to risk assessment:

- The use of systems biology to understand the different metabolic pathways that benzene interferes with to cause disease can help identify robust biomarkers of exposure, early effect, susceptibility, and disease development (Zhang et al., 2010). Combining tools from systems biology with large toxicogenomics databases might also improve these aspects in relation to other chemical exposures (McHale et al., 2010).

- A simplified model has been developed from animal and human data to predict blood levels of acrylonitrile from low levels of exposure (Takano et al., 2010).

The potential importance of the exposome in understanding better how chemicals such as organotins, perfluorooctanoic acid, phthalates, and bisphenol A (BFA) may disrupt hormones is discussed in relation to obesity and other metabolic disorders (Schnoor, 2011; Slomko et al., 2012). A comparison of different analytical approaches includes reference to an investigation into type 2 diabetes, and considers the methodological issues that arise (Thomas et al., 2012).

There are studies based on information on pre-natal exposures. Examples include: an investigation into pre-natal exposure to organo-chlorine compounds (Buck Louis et al., 2011); the use of proteomics to estimate foetal exposures and risk of chorioamnionitis (Buhimschi and Buhimschi, 2012); and epigenetic factors that may contribute to musculo-skeletal defects (Burwell et al., 2011). The ability to gather information on early (pre-natal) exposures was demonstrated as part of an investigation into persistent environmental chemicals, lifestyle, and fertility (Buck Louis et al., 2010).

Martien et al. (2011) proposes that a broader, multi-disciplinary approach is needed to translate research into improvements for patients with serious neurological disorders, who could benefit from identification and understanding of the exposome.

A review of papers on environmental risks for cancer also highlights the importance of transparency in defining what environment means, as there is a wide range of definitions used by different researchers (McGuinn et al., 2012). The use of antioxidants to reduce cancer risk is examined and it is suggested that more substances could be evaluated more rapidly if biomarkers of disease were developed that could identify cancer at an earlier stage (Goodman et al., 2011).

Genomics has provided limited progress towards reducing the burden of chronic conditions such as cancer, diabetes, obesity, heart disease, and neurological disorders. There is a growing desire to work across disciplines to produce tools that capture as many environmental stressors as possible that might interact with certain genetic traits to cause illness, noting that exposure to stressors will be extremely variable across time. This could create vast amounts of data, which would be extremely challenging to translate into meaningful information and interventions to protect and improve health. A collaborative approach will be needed to maximise the opportunities and minimise the risks associated with these advances. Most of these developments are likely to be driven by private companies and research institutes, and it will be important for public health bodies to maintain awareness of activity in this area.

Endocrine disrupting chemicals (EDCs)

Over the last decade, the scientific understanding of the relationship between exposure to endocrine disruptors and health has advanced rapidly. There is a growing concern that maternal, foetal, and childhood exposure to EDCs could play a larger role in the causation of many endocrine diseases and disorders than previously believed.

All species depend on the ability to reproduce and develop normally. This is not possible without a healthy endocrine system, the collection of glands in the body that secretes a range of hormones with a wide range of effects including regulating metabolism, growth and development, and sexual and reproductive functions. Almost every organ and cell in the body is influenced by, or dependent, on the endocrine system. An 'endocrine disruptor' is commonly defined as an exogenous substance or mixture that alters the function(s) of the endocrine system and consequently causes adverse health effects in an intact organism, or its progeny or (sub) populations (IPCS, 2002).

The potential impact of EDCs on human health came to prominence in the late 1990s, due to suggestions of a possible link between environmental chemical pollution and adverse effects on the male and female reproductive systems within wildlife (IEH, 1995). The initial evidence clearly identified various reproductive abnormalities suggestive of endocrine disruption, although generally these were in areas of elevated exposure to the relevant chemicals (IEH, 1999; IPCS, 2002). The effects in populations exposed to lower levels remained uncertain and the mechanisms for the adverse effects are not well understood.

Endocrine effects may be caused by a variety of chemicals leading to a range of effects and endocrine endpoints. Numerous chemicals have been identified as potential EDCs, including ones that are widely used, for example in personal care products, plasticisers, flame-retardants, pesticides, and pharmaceuticals. In 2002, an assessment of chemicals purported to be endocrine disruptors identified 966 potential compounds or elements, although the report noted that there were factual errors or inconsistencies within the source data (IEH, 2005).

Since then, intensive research has been undertaken to fill the data gaps and improve understanding of the impacts of EDCs (IPCS, 2013). One of the main drivers has been the rise in endocrine-related disease and disorders, for example, decreases in semen quality in young men and increases in endocrine-related cancers such as breast, prostate, and ovarian cancers, as well as increases in obesity and diabetes. Another important driver is that few of the chemicals currently in use (and their associated breakdown products) have been adequately studied for their endocrine disruption potential.

The *State of the Science of Endocrine Disrupting Chemicals 2012* report (IPCS, 2013) highlights a number of further areas of concern. Internationally agreed and validated testing procedures for the effects of EDCs capture only a limited range of the known spectrum of endocrine disrupting effects, which increases the likelihood that harmful effects in humans may be overlooked. Therefore, the disease risk due to EDCs may be underestimated and there is growing concern over maternal and foetal exposure to EDCs, as the time of exposure may be critical, especially in developing foetuses (IPCS, 2013).

EDCs are identified as an emerging issue by the Strategic Approach to International Chemicals Management (SAICM), which is a multi-sectoral policy framework intended to foster the sound management of chemicals. It recognises the goal agreed by the World Summit on Sustainable Development of ensuring that, by the year 2020, chemicals are produced and used in ways that minimise significant adverse impacts on the environment and human health. The SAICM have proposed a plan of action to address a number of priorities in relation to EDCs, which include assessing population groups with specific vulnerabilities, prioritising assessment of classes of chemicals that pose an unreasonable risk to human health and the environment (especially those that may adversely affect the endocrine system), and harmonising the methods for risk assessment and specific toxicological endpoints for endocrine disruption.

Summary

This chapter has highlighted the wide range of environmental factors that can significantly impact public health. The environment has been recognised as an important contributory factor to the overall burden of disease, and the speed with which the increases in disease incidence have occurred over recent decades cannot be simply ascribed to genetic factors as the sole plausible explanation. Environmental and other non-genetic factors, including nutrition, age of mother, and communicable disease history, are also linked to health in ways that may be difficult to identify, but some have been defined by research (IPCS, 2013).

It is important to recognise that the increasing production and use of chemicals, especially in developing regions of the world, may result in benefits for society, but the potential risks need to be assessed and balanced against the costs to human health, the environment, and sustainable development. Recognition of the importance of the impact of environmental factors in public health, whether when tackling inequalities or integrating environmental sustainability into public health interventions, has the potential to provide significant co-benefits across a range of outcomes.

The ability to accurately assess the impacts of environmental factors on health is rapidly improving through research and the identification of relevant indicators, which enable the use of common assessment frameworks to quantify the burden of disease attributable to the environment. These novel tools and frameworks, such as horizon scanning or the 'exposome', may be able to assist in identifying the interventions that have the potential to deliver maximum benefits, or in identifying future threats earlier.

References

Betts, K. S. (2011). A study in balance: How microbiomes are changing the shape of environmental health. *Environmental Health Perspectives*, **119**, a340–a346.

Birnbaum, L. S. (2010). Applying research to public health questions: Biologically relevant exposures. *Environmental Health Perspectives*, **118**:4, A152.

Bolte, G., Tamburlini, G., and Kohlhuber, M. (2010). Environmental inequalities among children in Europe: Evaluation of scientific evidence and policy implications. *European Journal of Public Health*, **20**:1, 14–20.

Buck Louis, G. M., Schisterman, E. F., Sweeney, A. M., et al. (2010). Preconception recruitment of couples desiring pregnancy—case for the exposome. *Fertility and Sterility*, **94**:4, S229.

Buck Louis, G. M., Schisterman, E. F., Sweeney, A. M., et al. (2011). Designing prospective cohort studies for assessing reproductive and developmental toxicity during sensitive windows of human reproduction and development: the Life Study. *Paediatric Perinatal Epidemiology*, **25**:5, 413–424.

Buhimschi, I. A. and Buhimschi, C. S. (2012). Proteomics/diagnosis of chorioamnionitis and of relationships with the fetal exposome. *Seminars in Fetal and Neonatal Medicine*, **17**:1, 36–45.

Burwell, R. G., Dangerfield, P. H., Moulton, A., and Grivas, T. B. (2011). Adolescent idiopathic scoliosis (AIS), environment, exposome, and epigenetics: A molecular perspective of postnatal normal spinal growth and the etiopathogenesis of AIS with consideration of a network approach and possible implications for medical therapy. *Scoliosis*, **6**:1, 26.

Committee for Science and Technology Challenges to US National Security Interests (2012). *Report of a Workshop on Big Data*. Available at: http://www.nap.edu/openbook.php?record_id=13541&page=R1 [Accessed 27 March 2013].

Corvalán, C. F., Kjellström, T., Smith, K. R. (1999). Health, environment and sustainable development. Identifying links and indicators to promote action. *Epidemiology*, **10**, 656–660.

Defra (2005). *The UK Government Sustainable Development Strategy*. Available at: https://www.gov.uk/government/uploads/system/uploads/attachment_data/file/69412/pb10589-securing-the-future-050307.pdf [Accessed 25 March 2013].

EU (2006). Renewed EU sustainable development strategy. 10917/06. (Adopted by the European Council 15/16 June 2006). Brussels. Available at: http://register.consilium.europa.eu/pdf/en/06/st10/st10117.en06.pdf [Accessed 25 March 2013].

Goodland, R. (1995). The concept of environmental sustainability. *Annual Review of Ecology and Systematics*, **26**, 1–24.

Goodman, M., Bostick, R. M., Kucuk, O., and Jones, D. P. (2011). Clinical trials of antioxidants as cancer prevention agents: Past, present, and future. *Free Radical Biology and Medicine*, **51**:5, 1068–1084.

Griffiths, J. (2006a). Mini-Symposium: Health and environmental sustainability. The convergence of public health and sustainable development. *Public Health*, **120**, 609–612.

Griffiths, J. (2006b). Environmental sustainability in the National Health Service in England. *Public Health*, **120**, 609–612.

Hamzelou, J. (2010). Want to know your disease risk? Check your exposome. *New Scientist* (Editorial), December. Available at: http://www.newscientist.com/article/mg20827921.800-want-to-know-your-disease-risk-check-your-exposome.html [Accessed 05 April 2013].

Hanninen, O. and Knol, A. (2011). European perspectives on environmental burden of disease. Estimates for nine stressors in six European countries. *European Perspectives on Environmental Burden of Disease Report 1*. Available at: http://www.thl.fi/thl-client/pdfs/b75f6999-e7c4-4550-a939-3bccb19e41c1 [Accessed 25 March 2013].

Horton, R. (2012). GBD 2010: Understanding disease, injury, and risk. *The Lancet*, **380**:9859, 2053–2054.

HPA (2005). *Health Protection in the 21st Century. Understanding the burden of disease: Preparing for the future*. Health Protection Agency. Available at: http://www.hpa.org.uk/webc/HPAwebFile/HPAweb_C/1194947403055 [Accessed 03 April 2013].

Human Genomics Strategy Group (2012). *Building on our Inheritance: Genomic technology in healthcare*. Available at: https://www.gov.uk/government/uploads/system/uploads/attachment_data/file/134568/dh_132382.pdf [Accessed 05 April 2013].

IEH (1995). IEH assessment on the environmental oestrogens: Consequences to human health and wildlife. *Institute for Environment and Health*. Available at: http://www.cranfield.ac.uk/about/people-and-resources/schools-and-departments/school-of-applied-sciences/groups-institutes-and-centres/ieh-reports-/endocrine-disruptors/a1.pdf [Accessed 09 April 2013].

IEH (1999). IEH assessment on the ecological significance of endocrine disruption: Effects on reproductive function and consequences for natural populations. *Institute for Environment and*

Health. Available at: http://www.cranfield.ac.uk/about/people-and-resources/schools-and-departments/school-of-applied-sciences/groups-institutes-and-centres/ieh-reports-/endocrine-disruptors/a4.pdf [Accessed 09 April 2013].

IEH (2005). Chemicals purported to be endocrine disruptors: A compilation of published lists (Web Report W20). *MRC Institute for Environment and Health*. Available at: http://www.cranfield.ac.uk/about/people-and-resources/schools-and-departments/school-of-applied-sciences/groups-institutes-and-centres/ieh-reports-/endocrine-disruptors/w20.pdf [Accessed 09 April 2013].

Institute for Health Metrics and Evaluation (2013). *The Global Burden of Disease: Generating Evidence, Guiding Policy*. Available at: http://www.healthmetricsandevaluation.org/sites/default/files/policy_report/2011/GBD_Generating%20Evidence_Guiding%20Policy%20FINAL.pdf [Accessed 25 March 2013].

IPCS (International Programme on Chemical Safety): Damstra, T., Barlow, S., Bergman, A., et al. (Eds) (2002). *Global Assessment of the State-of-the-science of Endocrine Disruptors*, WHO/PCS/EDC/02.2. Available at: http://www.who.int/ipcs/publications/new_issues/endocrine_disruptors/en/ [Accessed 09 April 2013].

IPCS (International Programme on Chemical Safety): Bergman, A., Heindel, J. J., Jobling, S., Kidd, K. A., and Zoeller, R. T. (Eds) (2013). *State of the Science of Endocrine-disrupting Chemicals 2012*. Available at: http://ehp.niehs.nih.gov/wp-content/uploads/121/4/ehp.1306695.pdf [Accessed 09 April 2013].

Lim, S. S., Vos, T., Flaxman, A. D., et al. (2012). The burden of disease and injury attributable to 67 risk factors and risk factor clusters in 21 regions 1990–2010: A systematic analysis. *Lancet*, **380**, 2224–2260.

Lioy, P. and Rappaport, S. M. (2011). Exposure science and the exposome: An opportunity for coherence in the environmental health sciences. *Environmental Health Perspectives*, **119**, 11.

Marmot, M. (Ed) (2010). *Fair Society, Healthy Lives: Strategic review of health inequalities in England post 2010*. Available at: http://www.instituteofhealthequity.org/projects/fair-society-healthy-lives-the-marmot-review [Accessed 25 March 2013].

Martien, J. H., Kas, V. K., Gould, T. D., et al (2011). Advances in multidisciplinary and cross-species approaches to examine the neurobiology of psychiatric disorders. *European Neuropsychopharmacology*, **21**:7, 532–544.

Martuzzi, M., Mitis, F., and Forastiere, F. (2010). Inequalities, inequities, environmental justice in waste management and health. *European Journal of Public Health*, **20**:1, 21–26.

Martyn, T., Smith, M. T., and Rappaport, S. M. (2009). Building exposure biology centers to put the E into 'G × E' interaction studies. *Environmental Health Perspectives*, **117**:8, A334–A335.

McGuinn, L. A., Ghazarian, A. A., Ellison, G. L., et al. (2012). Cancer and environment: Definitions and misconceptions. *Environmental Research*, **112**, 230–234.

McHale, C. M., Zhang, L., Hubbard, A. E., et al. (2010). Toxicogenomic profiling of chemically exposed humans in risk assessment. *Mutation Research/Reviews in Mutation Research*, **705**:3, 172–183.

McMichael, A. J., Campbell-Lendrum, D., Kovats, S., et al. (2003). Global climate change. In: Ezatti, M., Lopez, A. D., Rodgers, A., and Murray, C. J. L. (Eds). *Comparative Quantification of Health Risks: Global and regional burden of disease due to selected major risk factors*. World Health Organization, Geneva, Switzerland.

Moldan, B., Janouskova, S., and Hak, T. (2012). How to understand and measure environmental sustainability: indicators and targets. *Ecological Indicators*, **17**, 4–13.

Morris, G. P., Beck, S. A., Hanlon, P., and Robertson, R. (2006). Getting strategic about the environment and health. *Public Health*, **120**, 889–907.

Murray, C., Richards, M. L., Newton, J. N., et al. (2013). UK health performance: Findings of the Global Burden of Disease Study 2010. *Lancet*, **381**:9871, 997–1020. Available at: http://dx.doi.org/10.1016/S0140-6736(13)60355-4 [Accessed 25 March 2013].

Peters, A., Hoek, G., and Katsouyanni, K. (2012). Understanding the link between environmental exposures and health: Does the exposome promise too much? *Journal of Epidemiology and Community Health*, **66**, 103–105.

Prüss-Üstün, A. and Corvalán, C. (2006). *Preventing Disease Through Healthy Environments: Towards an estimate of the environmental burden of disease*. Available at: http://www.who.int/quantifying_ehimpacts/publications/preventingdisease.pdf [Accessed 03 April 2013].

Rappaport, S. M. (2012). Discovering environmental causes of disease. *Journal of Epidemiology and Community Health*, **66**, 99–102.

Schnoor, J. L. (2011). Obesogens, the exposome, and ES&T. *Environmental Science and Technology*, **45**:7, 2517.

Slomko, H., Heo, H. J., and Francine, H. (2012). Minireview: Epigenetics of obesity and diabetes in humans. *Endocrinology*, **153**:3, 1025–1030.

Takano, R., Murayama, N., Kana Horiuchi, K., et al. (2010). Blood concentrations of acrylonitrile in humans after oral administration extrapolated from in vivo rat pharmacokinetics, in vitro human metabolism, and physiologically based pharmacokinetic modelling. *Regulatory Toxicology and Pharmacology*, **58**:2, 252–258.

Thomas, D. C., Lewinger, J. P., Murcray, C. E., et al. (2012). Invited commentary: GE-Whiz! Ratcheting gene-environment studies up to the whole genome and the whole exposome. *American Journal of Epidemiology*, **175**:3, 203–207.

Traynor, B. J. and Singleton, A. B. (2010). Nature versus nurture: Death of a dogma, and the road ahead. *Neuron*, **68**:2, 196–200.

UN-HABITAT (2012). *State of the World's Cities 2012/13: Prosperity of cities*. Available at: http://www.unhabitat.org/pmss/listItemDetails.aspx?publicationID=3387 [Accessed 25 March 2013].

Vardoulakis, S. and Heaviside, C. (Eds) (2012). *Health Effects of Climate Change in the UK 2012: Current evidence, recommendations and research gaps*. Health Protection Agency. Centre for Radiation, Chemical and Environmental Hazards, UK. Available at: http://www.hpa.org.uk/hecc2012 [Accessed 07 June 2013].

WHO (2008). *Closing the Gap in a Generation: Health equity through action on the social determinants of health*. World Health Organization. Available at: http://whqlibdoc.who.int/publications/2008/9789241563703_eng.pdf [Accessed 25 March 2013].

WHO (2012). *Environmental Health Inequalities in Europe*. World Health Organization. Available at: http://www.euro.who.int/en/what-we-publish/abstracts/environmental-health-inequalities-in-europe.-assessment-report [Accessed 26 March 2013].

WHO (2013). *European Environment and Health Information System (ENHIS)*. World Health Organization. Available at: http://data.euro.who.int/eceh-enhis/Default2.aspx [Accessed 25 March 2013].

Wild, C. P. (2005). Complementing the genome with an 'exposome': The outstanding challenge of environmental exposure measurement in molecular epidemiology. *Cancer Epidemiology, Biomarkers and Prevention*, **14**: 8, 1847–1850.

Wild, C. P. (2011). Future research perspectives on environment and health: The requirement for a more expansive concept of translational cancer research. *Environmental Health*, **10**:Suppl 1, S15.

Wild, C. P. (2012). The exposome: From concept to utility. *International Journal of Epidemiology*, **41**:1, 24–32.

Zhang, L., McHale, C. M., Rothman, N., et al. (2010). Systems biology of human benzene exposure. *Chemico-Biological Interactions*, **184**:1–2, 86–93.

Further Reading

Environment and Health Information System (ENHIS) (2012). Available at: http://www.enhis.org/ [Accessed 07 June 2013].

European Community Health Indicators (ECHI) (2012). Available at: http://ec.europa.eu/health/indicators/echi/index_en.htm [Accessed 07 June 2013].

Strategic Approach to International Chemicals Management (SAICM) (2012). Available at: http://www.saicm.org/ [Accessed 07 June 2013].

UNIPHE (2012). *Use of Sub-National Indicators to Improve Public Health in Europe (UNIPHE)*. Available at: http://www.uniphe.eu/ [Accessed 07 June 2013].

Index of Statutes

A
Air Quality Directive (808/779/EEC) 59
Air Quality (England)(Amendment) Regulations (2002) 59
Air Quality (England) Regulations (2000) 59, 64
Air Quality Standards Regulations (2010) 59
Ambient Air Quality Directive (1999/30/EC) 59
Ambient Air Quality Directive (2008/50/EC) 59

C
Civil Contingencies Act (2004) 29
Clean Air Act (1956) 59
Clean Air Act (1968) 59
Clean Air Act (1993) 59
Control of Major Accident Hazards Regulations (1999) 26
Control of Pollution Act (1974) 118, 148

D
Deposit of Poisonous Waste Act (1972) 147
Drinking Water Directive (1998) 91–2

E
Environment Act (1995) 23, 25
  air pollution 60
  waste management 148, 151
Environmental Permitting (England and Wales) (Amendment) Regulations (2013) 24
Environmental Permitting Regulations (2010) 24, 27
  air pollution 63
  contaminated land 124
  waste management 149, 150, 151, 160, 164, 166, 169, 170
Environmental Protection Act (1990) 23
  contaminated land 118, 119, 120–3, 129, 130
  waste management 148, 151, 153, 160
  water 104–5
Environment (Northern Ireland) Order (2002) 60

F
Fourth Daughter Directive (2004/107/EC) 59

H
Hazardous Waste Directive 154
Health and Safety at Work Act (1974) 26
Health and Social Care Bill 26

I
Industrial Emissions Directive (2010/75/EU) 24, 63, 149, 150
Integrated Pollution Prevention and Control Directive (96/61/EC) 24
International Health Regulations (2005) 26

L
Landfill Directive (1993/31/EC) 149–50
Landfill Directive (1999) 160, 170
Landfill Regulations (2002) 148

N
National Emission Ceilings Directive (2001/81/EC) 58
National Emission Ceilings Regulations (2002) 58

P
Pollution Prevention Control Act (1999) 24
Pollution Prevention and Control Regulations (2000) 148
Private Water Supplies (England) Regulations (2009) 92
Private Water Supplies (Northern Ireland) Regulations (2009) 91
Private Water Supplies (Scotland) Regulations (2006) 93
Private Water Supplies (Wales) Regulations (2010) 92
Public Health Act (1848) 23
Public Health Act (1875) 23, 147
Public Health Act (1936) 23, 147
Public Health Act (1984) 26
Public Health (Control of Diseases) Act (1984) 26

R
Registration, Evaluation, Authorisation and restriction of Chemicals (REACH) Regulation (1907/2006) 26

S
Special Waste Regulations (1992) 148

T
Town and Country Planning Act (1990) 118, 120
Town and Country Planning Act (2010) 119–20

W
Waste (England and Wales) Regulations (2011) 148
Waste Framework Directive (75/442/EEC) 148–9, 154–6
Waste Framework Directive (2008/98/EC) 147, 148, 152
Waste (Household Waste Duty of Care)(England and Wales) Regulations (2005) 151
Waste Incineration Directive (2000/76/EC) 150–1, 164, 166, 167–8
Waste Management Licensing Regulations (1994) 148

INDEX OF STATUTES

Waste Management Licensing Regulations (2006) 105
Water Act (2003) 23, 91, 92
Water Framework Directive (2000) 93
Water Industry Act (1991) 23, 91, 92
Water Industry Act (1999) 23
Water (Northern Ireland) Order (1999) 93
Water Resources Act (1991) 23
Water (Scotland) Act (1980) 91
Water Supply (Domestic Distribution Systems) (Northern Ireland) Regulations (2009) 91
Water Supply (Water Quality)(Northern Ireland) Regulations (2007) 91
Water Supply (Water Quality) Regulations (2000) 92
Water Supply (Water Quality) Regulations (2001) 92
Water Supply (Water Quality)(Scotland) Regulations (2001) 91

Subject Index

A

Absolute Entries 154
abstraction licences 93
acceptable daily intake (ADI) 107–8
acrylonitrile 191
Action Plan 62, 63
Advanced Thermal Treatment (ATT) 165–7
air pollution and public health 3, 4, 57–86, 177, 179
   air pollution control (APC) chemicals 165
   air quality 18
      for London 2012 Olympics (case study) 71–2
      monitoring 63–4
   ambient air, impact of on health 64–6
   benzene 72
   Bonfire night 2007 (case study) 67
   1,3-butadiene 73
   carbon monoxide (CO) 73, 75
   Daily Air Quality Index (DAQI) 77–8
   Formaldehyde (case study) 74
   health effects pyramid 75–6
   incidents and emerging issues 83–6
      climate change 85–6
      fires and pollution 83–5
      ultrafine particulate matter 85
      waste tyre fire (case study) 84
   indoor air monitoring 74–5, 130
   intervention services 82
   lead 73
   legislation 58–63
      current 59–60
      environmental permitting 63
      historical background 58–9
      local air quality management (LAQM) 60–2
      London smog (case study) 58–9
      national air quality objectives 61
      spatial planning 62–3
   management areas (AQMAs) 62, 63, 69, 79
   mathematical modelling 48
   mitigation measures 78–83
      alerting and awareness raising (case study) 82
      emission reduction schemes: low emission zones 79–81
      individual intervention measures 81–2
      London Low Emission Zone (case study) 80–1
      pollutant removal from ambient air 81
      vehicles, alternatives to use of 82–3
   nitrogen dioxide (NO_2) 69–70
   ozone 70–2
   particulate matter 66–9
   Polycyclic Aromatic Hydrocarbons (PAHs) 73–4
   public health indicator 76–7
   sulfur dioxide (SO_2) 72
airTEXT service 82
aldrin 99–100
aluminium 94
ammonia (NH_3) 58
Anaerobic Digestion (AD) 162–3
analytical techniques 52–3, 54
aromatic hydrocarbons 117
   see also polycyclic aromatic hydrocarbons
arsenic 48, 94–5
asbestos 3, 139
as low as reasonably practicable (ALARP) principle 132
asthma 65, 69, 71, 72, 81, 82
Automatic Urban and Rural Network (AURN) 63–4

B

Benchmark Dose (BMD) 131–2
benzene 61, 64, 72, 130, 190–1
benzo(a)pyrene (BaP) 130
Best Available Techniques (BAT) 62, 63, 151, 164
Bhopal disaster (India) 36
bioaerosols 163–4
biomarkers of effect and exposure 138
biomass, thermal treatment of 167–8
birth defects and foetal exposure 161, 170, 192
black smoke 63–4
Bonfire night 2007 (case study) 67
boron 95
British Geological Survey (BGS) 48, 116, 125
Brundtland Commission 157
Bunker Hill, Idaho, USA (case study) 134
1,3-butadiene 61, 64, 73

C

carbetamide contamination (case study) 108
carbon dioxide (CO_2) 153, 164, 167
carbon monoxide (CO) 22, 61, 64, 73, 186
   indoor air quality 74–5
   poisoning (case study) 75
carcinogens and cancer 179
cardiovascular disorders/disease 66, 68–9, 73, 82, 85, 179, 183
Care4Air 82
cement production, alternative fuels, used for (case study) 170–1
Centre for Radiation, Chemical and Environmental Hazards (CRCE) 108–9, 110–11
Chemical Abstract Service (CAS) 9
Chemical Meteorology (CHEMET) 46–7
children and vulnerability to environmental hazards 2, 186
chlorinated aliphatic/aromatic hydrocarbons 117
chlorination 101, 102
chronic effect 133

Chronic obstructive pulmonary disease (COPD) 65–6, 72
climate change 85–6, 183–5
clopyralid 100
cluster identification 42
cohort studies 65
Combined Heat and Power (CHP) 167
Committee on carcinogenicity of chemicals in food, consumer products and the environment (COC) 164–5
Committee on the Medical Effects of Air Pollutants (COMEAP) 69, 74, 77, 171
Committee on toxicity of chemicals in food, consumer products and the environment (COT) 161
competent authority 28–9
composting 163–4
conceptual models 32–4, 126–7
contaminant 119
  linkages 126–7
  -pathway-receptor relationships 142
Contaminated Land Exposure Assessment (CLEA) 49, 128, 130, 135
contaminated land and public health 48–9, 115–43
  brownfield land 119
  contaminants associated with specific industries 118
  copper mine (case study) 137–8
  exposure assessment 133–8
    Bunker Hill, Idaho, USA (case study) 134
    dermal contact 135
    ingestion 134–5
    inhalation 135
    unusual routes 135–6
  inorganic contaminants 117
  lead mining (case study) 137
  legislation and legal framework 118–23
    Environmental Protection Act (1990) 120–3
    Town and Country Planning Act (2010) 119–20
  mitigating factors 136–8
  organic contaminants 117
  redevelopment of land introducing pathways to human health (case study) 120
  remediation and off-site issues 141–2
  risk assessment 125–32
    example (case study) 130–1
  risk communication 139–41
  roles and responsibilities 123–5
    Defra (Department for Environment, Food and Rural Affairs) 124–5
    Environment Agency (EA) 124
    local authorities 123–4
    public health professionals 125
    site developers/site owners 125
  sand gravel pit (case study) 141
  tar works (case study) 142
  toxicological aspects 131–2
Control of Major Accident Hazards (COMAH) regulations 28–9, 48
Control of Substances Hazardous to Health (COSHH) assessment 53

Convention on Long-Range Transboundary Air Pollution (CLRTAP) 58
copper 95–6, 137–8

D

Daily Air Quality Index 71, 82
decontamination ('clean up') techniques 9–10, 17, 18
Defra (Department for Environment, Food and Rural Affairs) 124–5
  Air Information Resource web pages 77
  contaminated land 120–3, 125
  environmental quality indicator 4
  London 2012 Olympics 71
  waste management 161, 163, 168, 170
  water 91
Department for Communities and Local Government 120
deprivation (socio-economic) 66
dermal contact 5, 10–11, 15, 17, 135
developmental effects and toxicity 4, 101, 109, 132, 133, 134
dieldrin 99–100
'dig and dump' (topsoil removal) 14, 142
dioxins 33–4, 139, 164, 168, 170
Directors of Public Health 25, 125
Disability-Adjusted Life Years (DALY) 2, 179–80, 181, 185
disease clusters 5
disinfection by products (DBPs) 101–2
dispersion modelling 3
DND (do not use for drinking or cooking) notice (water) 105–6
DNU (do not use for drinking, cooking or washing) notice (water) 105–6
dose-response assessment 5, 36
dot distribution mapping 43
DPSEEA model 177–8, 186–7
Drinking Water Inspectorate (DWI) 25, 91, 92–3
Drinking Water Quality Regulator (DWQR) 93
Duty of Care 151

E

2-EDD 110
2-EMD 110
emergency preparedness 48
emerging issues 175–93
  endocrine disrupting chemicals (EDCs) 191–3
  environmental inequalities 185–7
  environmental sustainability 181–5
  exposome study 189–91
  global burden of disease 178–81
  horizon scanning 188–9
  sub-national indicators to improve public health in Europe (case study) 187
emission limit values (ELVs) 63
endocrine disrupting chemicals (EDCs) 191–3
end-of-waste criteria 148
Environment Act (1995) 23
Environment Agency (EA) 25, 27, 28
  composting 164
  contaminated land 123, 124, 125, 126, 128, 141

Environment Agency (EA) (*continued*)
  environmental permitting and air quality 63
  hazardous waste 154
  landfill 160
  Soil and Herbage Pollutant Survey (2007) 22
  waste management 169, 170
  water 91, 92, 93
Environmental Action Programmes (EAPs) 148
environmental health (definition) 21
environmental inequalities 4, 185–7
environmental pathways 177
environmental permits 27–8, 170
environmental permitting and air quality 63
Environmental Protection Act (1990) 23, 120–3, 151
environmental science (definition) 21
environmental sustainability 181–5
  climate change (case study) 183–5
Environment and Health Information Systems (ENHIS) 186–7
epidemiological studies 4–6, 65
established thermal treatment: incineration 164–5
European Burden of Disease in Europe project (EBoDE) 180
European Food Safety Authority (EFSA) 108, 109
European Union:
  air quality 48, 58–60
  legislation 24
    standards and guidelines: development and use 60
    see also under waste management and public health
  nitrogen dioxide (NO2) 69
  particulate matter 68
  sub-national indicators to improve public health 187
  sustainability 182
European Waste Catalogue (EWC) 154
European Waste Framework (WFD) Directive 154–6
exposome study 189–91
exposure assessment *see under* contaminated land and public health
exposure modelling 138
exposure routes for humans 10

F
fires and pollution 83–5
flammable chemicals 13, 17, 155
Food Standards Agency (FSA) 26, 125
formaldehyde levels, elevated (case study) 74
framework for investigation *see* key concepts and framework for investigation

G
gases 10–11
gasification 165–6
Generic Assessment Criteria (GAC) 127–8, 130, 132, 139
geocoding 42
geographic information system (GIS) 5, 39–43, 46, 48, 52
  analysis 39

  basic tools 41
  benefits 43, 49
  complex tools 41–2
  data 39–41
  display 39
  limitations 49–50
  types of mapping 42–3
global burden of disease 178–81
global positioning systems (GPS) 38
Gothenburg Protocol 58
government bodies and regulatory authorities 25–6
granular activated carbon (GAC) 102

H
half-life *see* persistence
haloacetic acids (HAAs) 101
hazard 1–2, 3, 30
  characterisation 35
  identification 35
  modern 176–7
  traditional 176–7
hazardous waste 157, 160
Health Criteria Value (HCV) 127–8, 131–2, 135, 139, 142
health protection 4–6
Health Protection Agency (HPA) 48
health and safety considerations 53
Health and Safety Executive (HSE) 26, 28
heavy metals 116
Henry's Law constant 10, 12
hexavalent chromium 52–3
horizon scanning 188–9
Human Genomics Strategy Group 189
hydrocarbons 117

I
incineration 159, 164–5
index dose (ID) 132
Industrial Emissions Directive (2010/75/EU) 150
Industrial Revolution 23
inert waste 157, 160
ingestion 5, 13, 14, 15, 18, 134–5
inhalation 5, 10, 11, 12, 13, 15, 17, 135
inorganic chemicals 16, 117
insoluble chemicals 15
Institute of Occupational Medicine 164
International Agency for Research on Cancer (IARC0) 100
iron 96

K
kerosene 15
key concepts and framework for investigation 20–55
  Control of Major Accident Hazards (COMAH) regulations 28–9
  definitions in environmental risk assessment 30
  environmental health (definition) 21
  environmental permitting 27–8
  environmental science (definition) 21
  government bodies and regulatory authorities in England and Wales 25–6

legislation 23–9
non-communicable disease, role of public health in 26–7
pollution sources 21–2
REACH (Registration, Evaluation, Authorisation and restriction of Chemicals 24
risk communication 37–8
risk perception 37–8
risk screening matrix 30
sampling and monitoring 50–4
sensitive receptors 22
Seveso, Italy accident (case study) 28
stakeholder and public participation and engagement 37–8
see also risk assessment

L
land *see* contaminated land
landfill 159–61
Landfill Directive (1993/31/EC) 149–50
latency of effects 139
Law Commission Law Reform Programme (Ninth) 26
lead 3, 59, 61, 73, 179
  contaminated land 116, 133, 134, 137
  contaminated water 97, 108–10
  legislation 23–4
  limits of detection (LOD) 53
limit values 60, 63
liquids 10
List of Waste 154
local air quality management (LAQM) 60–2, 63
local authorities 25, 27
  air quality 63
  contaminated land 123–4, 125, 141
  waste management 169–70
Local Industry Forum 62
Local Planning Authority 119–20, 123–4
London Air Quality Network (LAQN) 64
London Low Emission Zone (case study) 80–1
London smog (case study) 58–9
low emission zones (LEZs) 79–81
Lowest Observed Adverse Effect Levels (LOAELs) 129

M
manganese 97–8
mapping 43
Marmott review 4
mathematical modelling 43–9
  advantages 49
  air quality 48
  arsenic assessment in Cornwall 48
  contaminated land 48–9
  emergency preparedness 48
  limitations 49–50
  monitoring and modelling 44–5
  proactive models 46, 48–9
  reactive models 46, 47
  traffic management 48

Mayor's Air Quality Strategy (MAQS) (London) 79–80
mean daily intake (MDI) 132
Mechanical Biological Treatment (MBT) 161–2
membrane filtration 102
mercury 15
mesophilic processes 162
metabolic disorders 96, 190–1
metaldehyde 100
metals 16, 117
  incineration 164
methaemoglobinaemia 98–9
Mirror Entries 154
molecular weight (MW) 10, 12, 17
monitoring *see* sampling and monitoring
morbidity 76, 179
mortality 2, 4, 176, 179
  air pollution 68–9, 71, 72, 75–6, 77
  heat- and cold-related 183–4
multi-agency group formation 140–1
multi-criteria decision analysis (MCDA) 37
municipal solid waste (MSW) 161–2, 164, 165

N
nanoparticles *see* ultrafine particulate matter
naphthalene 142
National Planning Policy Framework (NPPF) 63
Natural Resources Wales 21, 25
  contaminated land 123
  landfill 160
  waste management 169
  water 92, 93
neurological effects and toxicity 73, 94, 98, 100, 191
neurotoxins 17
nitrate and nitrite 98–9
nitric oxide (NO) 22, 69–70
nitrogen dioxide (NO_2) 22, 59, 61, 62, 63, 64, 69–70
  air pollution mitigation measures 79, 81
  gaseous waste management 153
  health burden and ambient air pollution 78
  indoor air quality 74
non-communicable disease, role of public health in 26–7
Non-Hazardous Entries 154
non-hazardous waste 157, 160
non-metals 117
no observed adverse effect level (NOAEL) 131
Normal Background Concentrations (NBC) 116, 118

O
objectives 60
off-site emergency plans 29
options appraisal 37
organic carbon-water partition coefficient (soil sorption) 14
organic chemicals 14, 16, 116
Organisation for Economic Cooperation and Development (OECD) environmental strategy 181
organometallics 117
organ-specific effects 133

orthophosphorous acid 102
oxides of nitrogen (NOx) 58, 59, 64, 68, 69–70
　air pollution mitigation measures 79–81
　biomass 168
　incineration 164
　and ozone, relationship between 70
ozonation 102
ozone (O3) 22, 61, 64, 70–2, 184
　air pollution mitigation measures 81
　climate change 85–6
　depletion 177
　health burden and ambient air pollution 71, 78
　sources 70–1, 72
　susceptible groups 65

P

particulate matter 3–4, 59, 63–4, 66–9, 181
　air pollution mitigation measures 79
　anthropogenic (primary or direct) 67
　biomass 168
　fires 84
　incineration 164
　natural sources 67
　$PM_{2.5}$ 60, 61, 64, 66, 67, 68–9, 85
　　biomass 168
　　health burden and ambient air pollution 75–6, 77, 78
　PM_{10} 61, 62, 64, 66, 67, 68–9, 85
　　air pollution mitigation measures 79, 81
　　biomass 167
　　health burden and ambient air pollution 78
　regional and national/international sources 68
　secondary sources 68
　ultrafine 66, 68, 85
perfluorooctane sulfonic acid (PFOS) 15
persistence (half-life in soil, air, water) 11, 14–15, 17
personal protective equipment (PPE) 53
pesticides 99–100
pH adjustment 102
physicochemical properties 9–18
　chemical partitioning 15–18
　exposure routes for humans 10
　interpretations 11–12, 17
　organic carbon-water partition coefficient (soil sorption) 14
　partition coefficient between water and octanol 14
　persistence (half-life in soil, air, water) 14–15
　physical form 10, 12, 17
　specific gravity 15
　vapour density 13
　vapour pressure 13
　waste fire (case study) 16–18
　water solubility 13–14
plume dispersion model 44–6
polluter pays principle 148
Pollution Prevention and Control Act (1999) 24
pollution sources 21–2
polycyclic aromatic hydrocarbons (PAHs) 61, 73–4
　biomass 168
　contaminated land 116, 130, 139
　incineration 164

pregnant women and susceptibility to harmful toxins 73, 95, 99, 101, 131, 134, 191, 192
　see also birth defects
primary pollutants 21–2
proactive models 46, 48–9
probabilities assessment 35–6
problem formulation 32–5
proportional symbols mapping 43
protein adduct analysis 190
psychological impacts 139
public exposure 17
Public Health England (PHE) 25, 125, 170
Public Health Outcomes Framework 77
public health professionals 125, 170–1
Public Health Wales (PHW) 26, 125
pyrolysis 165–6

Q

qualitative analysis 35, 36, 126
quality control (QC) 52–3
quality of the environment 1
quantitative analysis 35, 36

R

REACH (Registration, Evaluation, Authorisation and restriction of Chemicals) 4, 24
receptors 22, 119
recycling 158–9, 160
regeneration 181
regulatory authorities 25–6
remote sensing 38
reproductive effects and toxicity 4, 95, 134, 192
respiratory disorders/diseases 66, 68–9, 71, 72, 81, 85
　climate change 183
　composting 164
　fires 84
　see also asthma; *Chronic obstructive pulmonary disease*
risk 1–2, 3
　coefficients 5
　communication 37–8, 139–41
　management 30
　perception 37–8, 171
　screening 35
　　matrix 30
　see also risk assessment
risk assessment 30–7
　event tree analysis 36
　geographic information system (GIS) 39–43
　hazard characterisation 35
　hazard identification 35
　mathematical modelling 43–9
　options appraisal 37
　prioritised risk 35
　probabilities assessment 35–6
　problem formulation 32–5
　soil contamination risk assessment (case study) 33–4
　tools 38–50
　and uncertainty characterisation 36–7
　water and public health 105–6

Risk Based Corrective Action (RBCA) 129
Risk Integrated Software for Clean-ups (RISC) 129

S

sampling and monitoring 3, 50–4
  air (indoor and outdoor) 50
  analytical and quality control considerations 52–3
  blind samples 53
  collection of samples 54
  duplicate sampling 53
  health and safety considerations 53
  planning 51–4
  sampling protocol 52
  sampling strategy 51–2
  soil and vegetation 51
  water environments 51
sand gravel pit (case study) 141
science, environmental 4–6
Scottish Environmental Protection Agency (SEPA) 28, 93, 123, 169
secondary pollutants 21–2
selenium 100–1
semi-metals 117
semi-quantitative analysis 35
sensitisation effects 133
Seveso Directive 28
Seveso, Italy accident (case study) 28
sewers 103
sheltering and fire 84–5
significant contaminant linkage 121
significant harm 121–3
significant possibility of significant harm (SHOSH) 22, 121, 130–1
site investigation 127
site-specific assessment criteria (SSAC) 129, 130
site-specific bioaerosol risk assessment (SSBRA) 164
sludge treatment and disposal 103–5
social media and communication of hazards 38
socio-economic factors 177, 179, 185–6
soil contamination risk assessment (case study) 33–4
Soil Guideline Values (SGVs) 128, 130, 131–2, 137, 139
soil sorption 12, 14, 17
soil and vegetation sampling and monitoring 51
source-pathway-receptor model 3, 33, 34
spatial planning and air quality 62–3
spatial statistics 42
'special sites' 123–4
speciation 16
specific gravity 12, 15
stakeholders and public participation and engagement 30, 32, 37–8
Standard Rules Environmental Permit 166
standards and guidelines:
  air quality 60
  quality control 53
  see also under water and public health
Strategic Approach to International Chemicals Management (SAICM) 192–3
sub-national indicators to improve public health in Europe (case study) 187

sulfur dioxide (SO2) 58, 59, 61, 62, 63–4, 72
  biomass 168
  fires 84
  gaseous waste management 153
  health burden and ambient air pollution 78
  incineration 164
  indoor air quality 74
  particulate matter 68
sulfur trioxide (SO_3) 168
susceptible groups 3, 77–8
  ambient air 65–6
  fires 84
  see also cardiovascular disorders/disease; children; pregnant women; respiratory disorders/diseases
syngas 165
systeic (whole body) effects 133

T

target values 60
tar materials 142, 166–7
temperature and vapour pressure 13
tetrachloro-dibenzo-para-dioxin (TCDD) 28
tetrachloroethylene 16, 17
thermal desorption of waste tar materials (case study) 166–7
thermal treatment of biomass 167–8
thermophilic processes 162
tolerable daily intake (TDI) 34, 107, 131–2, 137
tolerable daily soil intake (TDSI) 132
Town and Country Planning Act (2010) 119–20
toxicodynamics 5
toxicokinetics 5
toxicological aspects 131–3
toxicology, environmental 4–6
toxic waste 155
trihalomethanes (THMs) 101
trivalent chromium 52–3
tyres 170

U

UK Accreditation Service laboratory 52
ultrafine particulate matter 66, 68, 85
ultraviolet (UV) radiation 102
uncertainty and risk assessment 30
United Nations General Assembly 90
Updating and Screening Assessment 61
Urban Heavy Metals Network 64

V

vapour density 11, 13, 17
vapour pressure (VP) 11, 13, 17
vehicles, alternatives to use of 82–3
ventilation 13, 17
volatile organic compounds (VOCs) 13, 16, 17, 58, 64, 68
  biomass 168
  contaminated land 130
  fires 84
  indoor air quality 74

volatile organic compounds (VOCs) (*continued*)
  ozone 70
  syngas 165
  waste management 163

W

waste-derived fuel (WDF) 170
waste fire (case study) 16–18
Waste Framework Directive (75/442/EEC) 148–9
waste hierarchy 158, 159
Waste Incineration Directive (WID)(2000/76/EC) 150–1
waste management licence 105
waste management and public health 146–72
  Advanced Thermal Treatment (ATT) 165–7
  anaerobic digestion (AD) 162–3
  cement production (case study) 170–1
  composting 163–4
  disposal 159–60
  environmental agencies 169
  Environmental Protection Act (1990) 151
  established thermal treatment: incineration 164–5
  European legislation 148–51
    Industrial Emissions Directive (2010/75/EU) 150
    Landfill Directive (1993/31/EC) 149–50
    Waste Framework Directive (75/442/EEC) 148–9, 154–6
    Waste Incineration Directive (WID)(2000/76/EC) 150–1
  importance of waste and concerns 146–7
  local authorities 169–70
  Mechanical Biological Treatment (MBT) 161–2
  modern landfill 160–1
  prevention measures 158
  public health professionals 170–1
  public health support to regulators at public meetings (case study) 171
  recovery 160
  recycling 158–9
  reuse 158, 160
  risk perception 171
  sensitising 155
  sources of controlled waste 156–7
  thermal desorption of waste tar materials (case study) 166–7
  thermal treatment of biomass 167–8
  unlicensed waste facility (case study) 150
  waste controlled under European Waste Framework (WFD) Directive: non-hazardous waste 156

  waste excluded from scope of Waste Framework Directive (WFD) 153
  waste hierarchy 148–9
water-based cleaning methods 14
Water Industry Act (1991) 23
Water Management Unit (WMU) 93
water and public health 18, 90–111, 177
  chemical pollutants 93–102
    aluminium 94
    arsenic 94–5
    boron 95
    copper 95–6
    disinfection by-products (DBPs) 101–2
    iron 96
    lead 97
    manganese 97–8
    nitrate and nitrite 98–9
    pesticides 99–100
    selenium 100–1
  Drinking Water Inspectorate (DWI) 91
  drinking water sources and treatment 102–5
    sludge treatment and disposal 103–5
    wastewater treatment and disposal 102–3
  fresh, marine, surface and underground water 93
  private water supplies 92–3
  public water supplies 92
  risk assessment 105–6
  sampling and monitoring 51
  standards and guidelines 106–11
    carbetamide contamination (case study) 108
    development 106–7
    intakes calculation from chemical exposure 107–11
    lead contamination (case study) 108–10
    unusual tastes and odours in drinking water (case study) 110–11
  wholesome water 91–2
Water Resources Act (1991) 23
water solubility 11, 13–14, 17
wet wiping 12
World Health Organization (WHO) 181
  air quality Guidelines 59, 71, 74
  arsenic 94–5
  Commission on Social Determinants of Health (CSDH) 185–6
  European Region 187
  iron 96
  water quality guidelines 90, 91, 107